SOMATIC

EXERCISES

FOR

NERVOUS

SYSTEM

REGULATION

Relieve Stress, Overcome Anxiety, and Calm Your Body with Guided Techniques and Practices for Daily Relief

Elizabeth C. Nicholson

Copyright © 2024 by Elizabeth C. Nicholson
All rights reserved. No part of this book may be reproduced, distributed, or transmitted in any form or by any means, including photocopying, recording, or other electronic or mechanical methods, without the prior written permission of the publisher, except in the case of brief quotations embodied in critical reviews and certain other noncommercial uses permitted by copyright law.

CONTENT

CONTENT

CONTENT

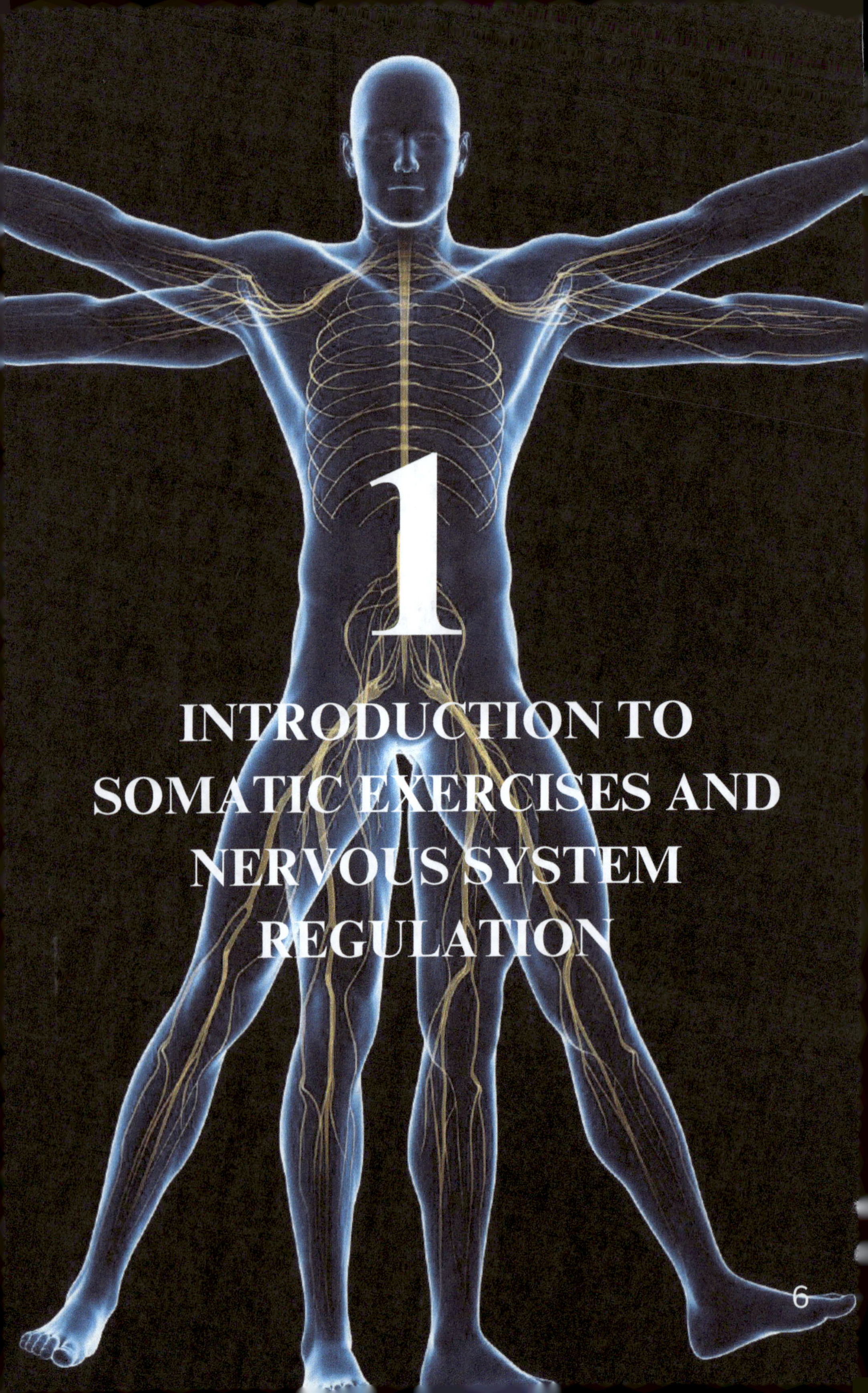

1

INTRODUCTION TO
SOMATIC EXERCISES AND
NERVOUS SYSTEM
REGULATION

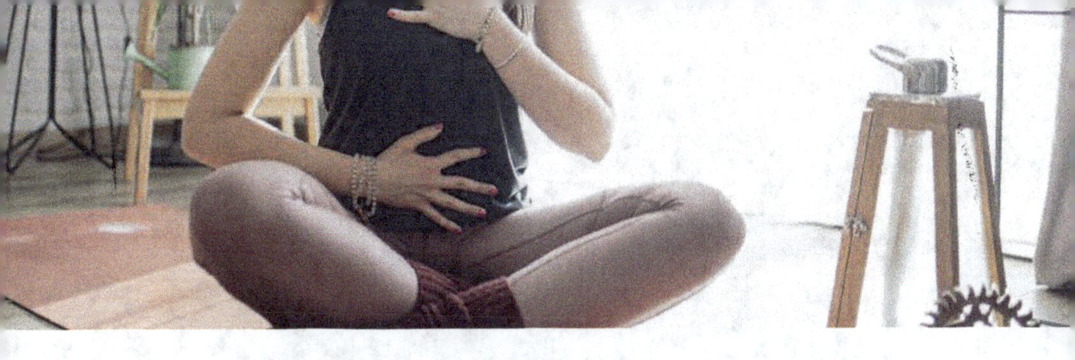

UNDERSTANDING SOMATIC EXERCISES

Somatic exercises are a holistic approach to body-mind integration, focusing on internal physical perception and experience. Unlike conventional fitness routines that emphasize external movements and muscle strength, somatic exercises prioritize the internal awareness of the body. These exercises help individuals develop a deeper connection with their physical selves, enabling them to sense, feel, and control their bodily movements more effectively.

Somatic exercises draw from various disciplines, including yoga, Pilates, Feldenkrais, and Alexander Technique. They involve gentle, mindful movements that are designed to release tension, improve posture, and enhance overall body awareness. By practicing somatic exercises regularly, individuals can achieve a greater sense of balance and harmony within their bodies.

THE IMPORTANCE OF NERVOUS SYSTEM REGULATION

The nervous system plays a crucial role in regulating bodily functions and maintaining overall health. It is responsible for controlling both voluntary and involuntary actions, such as movement, sensation, and autonomic functions like heart rate and digestion. The nervous system is divided into two main parts: the central nervous system (CNS), comprising the brain and spinal cord, and the peripheral nervous system (PNS), which includes all the nerves outside the CNS.

Regulating the nervous system is essential for managing stress, anxiety, and emotional well-being. Chronic stress and trauma can dysregulate the nervous system, leading to various physical and mental health issues. Symptoms of a dysregulated nervous system include chronic pain, fatigue, digestive problems, and mood disorders. By practicing somatic exercises, individuals can help restore balance to their nervous system, promoting overall health and well-being.

HOW SOMATIC EXERCISES WORK

Somatic exercises work by enhancing the body's natural ability to self-regulate and heal. These exercises focus on slow, mindful movements that encourage individuals to pay close attention to their bodily sensations. This heightened awareness helps identify and release areas of tension and discomfort, leading to improved movement patterns and greater ease in daily activities.

One key aspect of somatic exercises is the activation of the parasympathetic nervous system, which is responsible for the body's rest-and-digest response. By engaging in gentle, calming movements, somatic exercises help shift the body from a state of stress (sympathetic dominance) to a state of relaxation and restoration (parasympathetic dominance). This shift promotes healing, reduces stress hormones, and supports overall health.

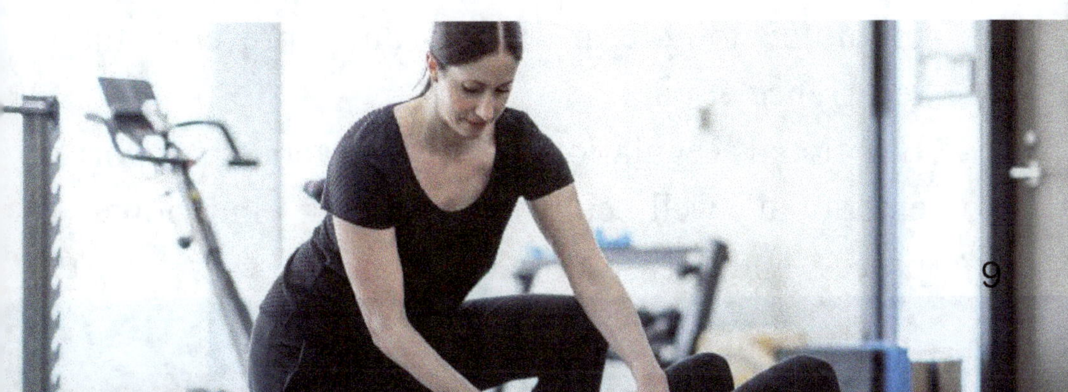

BENEFITS OF INCORPORATING SOMATIC PRACTICES

Incorporating somatic practices into your daily routine can provide numerous benefits, both physically and mentally. Some of the key benefits include:

1. Stress Reduction: Somatic exercises help calm the nervous system, reducing the physical and mental effects of stress. This can lead to improved mood, better sleep, and increased resilience to daily challenges.

2. Improved Body Awareness: By focusing on internal sensations and movements, individuals develop a deeper connection with their bodies. This heightened awareness can improve posture, coordination, and overall physical functioning.

3. Pain Relief: Somatic exercises can help release chronic tension and alleviate pain. By addressing the root causes of discomfort, these exercises promote long-term relief and prevent the recurrence of pain.

4. Emotional Regulation: Somatic practices support emotional well-being by helping individuals process and release stored emotions.

This can lead to greater emotional resilience and a more balanced mood.

5. Enhanced Relaxation: The gentle, mindful movements of somatic exercises promote relaxation and reduce the activation of the body's stress response. This can improve sleep quality and overall sense of calm.

6. Holistic Healing: Somatic exercises address the interconnectedness of the body and mind, promoting holistic healing and well-being. By supporting the body's natural healing processes, these practices can lead to improved health and vitality.

Incorporating somatic exercises into your routine can transform your relationship with your body and mind. As you progress through this book, you will discover various techniques and practices that will help you achieve a balanced and regulated nervous system, leading to a healthier, happier, and more fulfilling life.

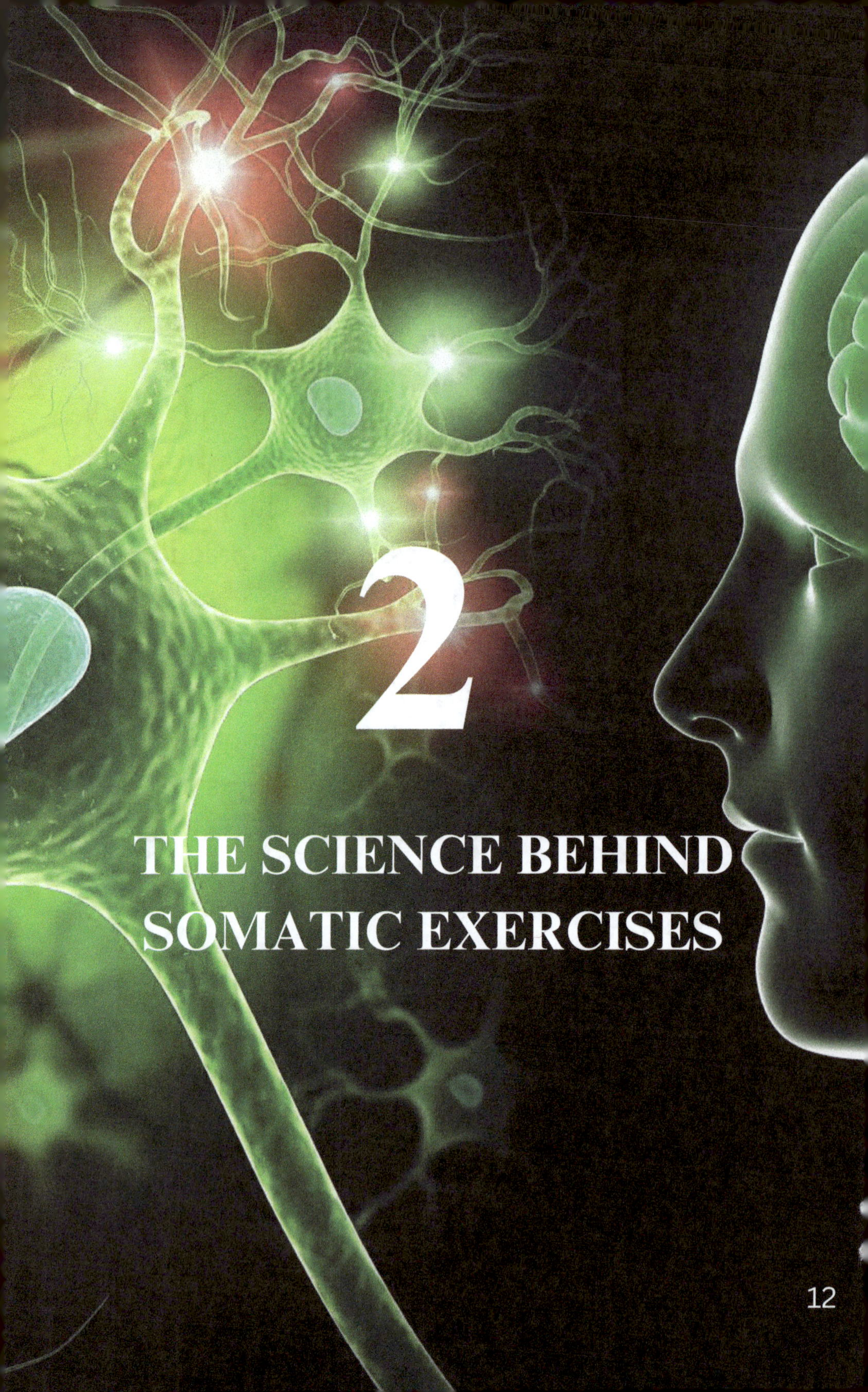
2
THE SCIENCE BEHIND
SOMATIC EXERCISES

THE ROLE OF THE NERVOUS SYSTEM

The nervous system is the body's command center, overseeing both voluntary and involuntary actions. It is divided into two main components: the central nervous system (CNS), comprising the brain and spinal cord, and the peripheral nervous system (PNS), which includes all the nerves outside the CNS. Together, these systems coordinate activities throughout the body, from muscle movements to hormone release.

1. Central Nervous System (CNS):
   - The CNS is responsible for processing sensory information and responding accordingly. The brain interprets input from the senses and makes decisions, while the spinal cord serves as a conduit for signals between the brain and the rest of the body. The CNS plays a pivotal role in maintaining homeostasis, ensuring that the body's internal environment remains stable despite external changes.
2. Peripheral Nervous System (PNS):
   - The **PNS** connects the CNS to limbs and organs.

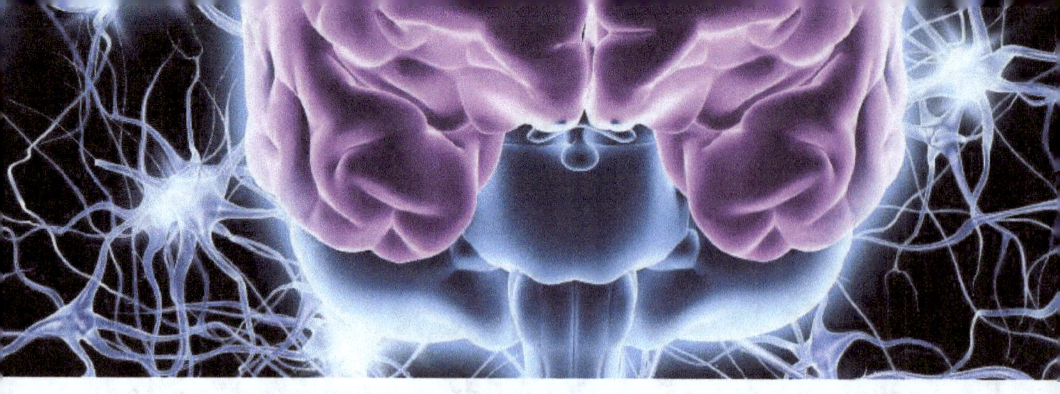

- It is further divided into the somatic nervous system, which controls voluntary movements, and the autonomic nervous system (ANS), which regulates involuntary functions such as heart rate, digestion, and respiratory rate. The ANS itself has two branches: the sympathetic nervous system, which prepares the body for action ('fight or flight'), and the parasympathetic nervous system, which calms the body and conserves energy ('rest and digest').

Understanding the complex interactions within the nervous system helps explain how somatic exercises can influence overall health. These exercises can recalibrate the balance between the sympathetic and parasympathetic systems, promoting a state of relaxation and recovery that is essential for health and well-being.

Vagus Nerve and Its Impact on Health

The vagus nerve, the longest cranial nerve in the body, is a critical component of the parasympathetic nervous system. It extends from the brainstem down through the neck and into the chest and abdomen, influencing the heart, lungs, and digestive tract. The vagus nerve plays a key role in regulating many bodily functions, making it integral to maintaining overall health.

1. Heart and Respiratory Regulation:
   - The vagus nerve helps regulate heart rate by sending signals that slow the heartbeat, promoting a calm and relaxed state. It also influences respiratory rate and patterns, encouraging deep, steady breathing that enhances oxygen exchange and reduces stress.
2. Digestive Health:
   - Vagal stimulation promotes digestion by increasing the secretion of digestive enzymes and enhancing gut motility. It also helps regulate the balance of gut microbiota, which is crucial for a healthy digestive system and immune function.
3. Inflammation Control:
   - The vagus nerve plays a role in

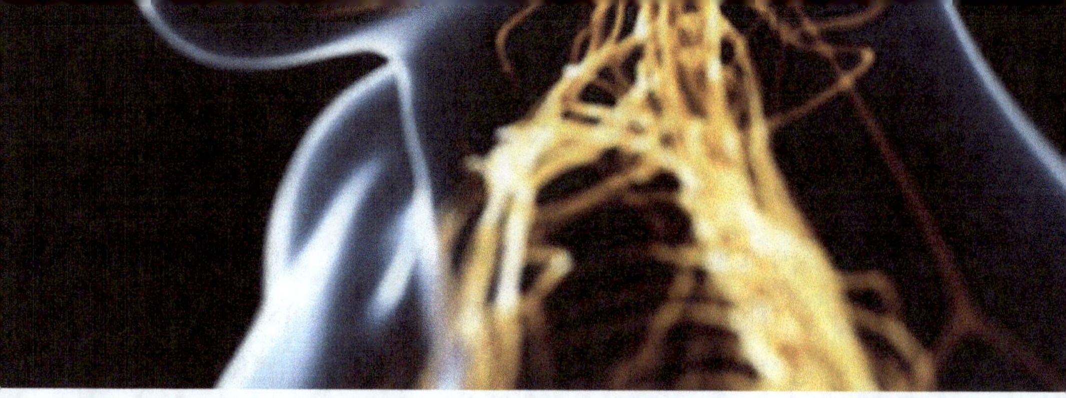

the inflammatory response. Vagal signals can suppress the production of pro-inflammatory cytokines, reducing inflammation and its harmful effects on the body. This anti-inflammatory effect is particularly beneficial for managing chronic conditions such as arthritis and autoimmune diseases.

- Emotional and Mental Health:
  - The vagus nerve is connected to the brain regions involved in emotion regulation and social bonding. Vagal tone, or the activity of the vagus nerve, has been linked to emotional resilience, stress response, and overall psychological well-being. Higher vagal tone is associated with a greater ability to manage stress and maintain emotional balance.

Somatic exercises can stimulate the vagus nerve, enhancing its beneficial effects on the body. Techniques such as deep breathing, gentle movements, and mindful practices activate the parasympathetic system, promoting relaxation and health.

STRESS AND TRAUMA: EFFECTS ON THE NERVOUS SYSTEM

Chronic stress and trauma can have profound effects on the nervous system, leading to dysregulation and various health issues. Understanding these effects is crucial for appreciating how somatic exercises can help restore balance and promote healing.

1. Chronic Stress:
   - When the body perceives a threat, the sympathetic nervous system activates the 'fight or flight' response, releasing stress hormones like adrenaline and cortisol. While this response is beneficial in short-term danger, chronic activation due to ongoing stress can have detrimental effects. Prolonged stress can lead to heightened arousal, anxiety, and an inability to relax, as well as physical symptoms like high blood pressure, digestive problems, and a weakened immune system.

2. Trauma:
   - Trauma, whether from a single event or prolonged exposure to adverse conditions, can deeply impact the nervous system.

- Traumatic experiences often leave individuals in a state of hyperarousal or dissociation, where the nervous system remains stuck in 'fight, flight, or freeze' modes. This can lead to chronic pain, emotional dysregulation, and conditions such as PTSD.

3. Nervous System Dysregulation:

- Dysregulation of the nervous system due to stress or trauma disrupts the balance between the sympathetic and parasympathetic systems. This imbalance can manifest as hypervigilance, insomnia, digestive issues, chronic fatigue, and other health problems. The body loses its ability to efficiently switch between states of arousal and relaxation, leading to persistent stress and health deterioration.

Somatic exercises help counteract the effects of stress and trauma by promoting nervous system regulation. These practices encourage a return to the parasympathetic state, facilitating recovery and healing.

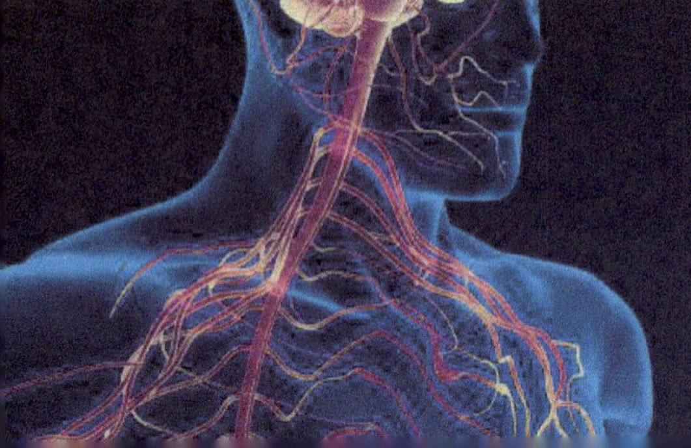

Scientific Evidence Supporting Somatic Practices

The efficacy of somatic exercises is supported by a growing body of scientific research. Studies demonstrate the positive impact of these practices on physical and mental health, providing a solid foundation for their use in nervous system regulation.

1. Stress Reduction and Relaxation:
   - Research shows that somatic practices, such as deep breathing, progressive muscle relaxation, and gentle movement exercises, significantly reduce stress levels. These practices lower cortisol levels, decrease heart rate, and promote a state of relaxation, which is beneficial for both mental and physical health.

2. Pain Management:
   - Somatic exercises have been found effective in managing chronic pain. Techniques like the Feldenkrais Method and Alexander Technique help improve body awareness and movement patterns, reducing pain and increasing mobility. Studies indicate that these methods can lead to long-term pain relief and improved quality of life for individuals with chronic pain conditions.

3. Emotional and Psychological Benefits:
   - Evidence supports the role of somatic practices in improving emotional regulation and mental health. Practices such as mindfulness, body scanning, and movement therapy have been shown to reduce symptoms of anxiety, depression, and PTSD. These exercises enhance emotional resilience and provide tools for coping with stress and trauma.
4. Neuroplasticity and Healing:
   - Somatic exercises promote neuroplasticity, the brain's ability to reorganize and form new neural connections. This is particularly important for healing from trauma and stress-related conditions. By engaging in mindful movement and body awareness practices, individuals can rewire their nervous systems, fostering recovery and resilience.
5. Enhancement of Vagal Tone:
   - Studies indicate that somatic practices can enhance vagal tone, improving the function of the vagus nerve and its regulatory effects on the body. Techniques such as deep breathing and gentle stretching stimulate vagal activity, promoting a state of calm and balance.

4. Improved Sleep Quality:
   - Research demonstrates that somatic exercises can improve sleep quality by promoting relaxation and reducing stress. Practices such as guided imagery and gentle stretching before bedtime help individuals transition into a restful state, enhancing sleep duration and quality.
5. Digestive Health:
   - Somatic practices positively impact digestive health by reducing stress and enhancing vagal activity. Techniques such as abdominal breathing and mindful eating improve digestion and gut motility, addressing issues like irritable bowel syndrome (IBS) and other stress-related digestive disorders.
6. Holistic Health and Well-being:
   - Overall, somatic exercises contribute to holistic health and well-being. By fostering a deep connection between the body and mind, these practices support physical health, emotional resilience, and psychological balance. They provide a comprehensive approach to maintaining and enhancing overall health.

Incorporating somatic exercises into daily life offers a scientifically supported method for regulating the nervous system and promoting overall health. These practices provide a powerful toolset for managing stress, healing from trauma, and achieving a balanced state of well-being. As you explore the techniques and principles in this book, you will discover how somatic exercises can transform your health and enrich your life.

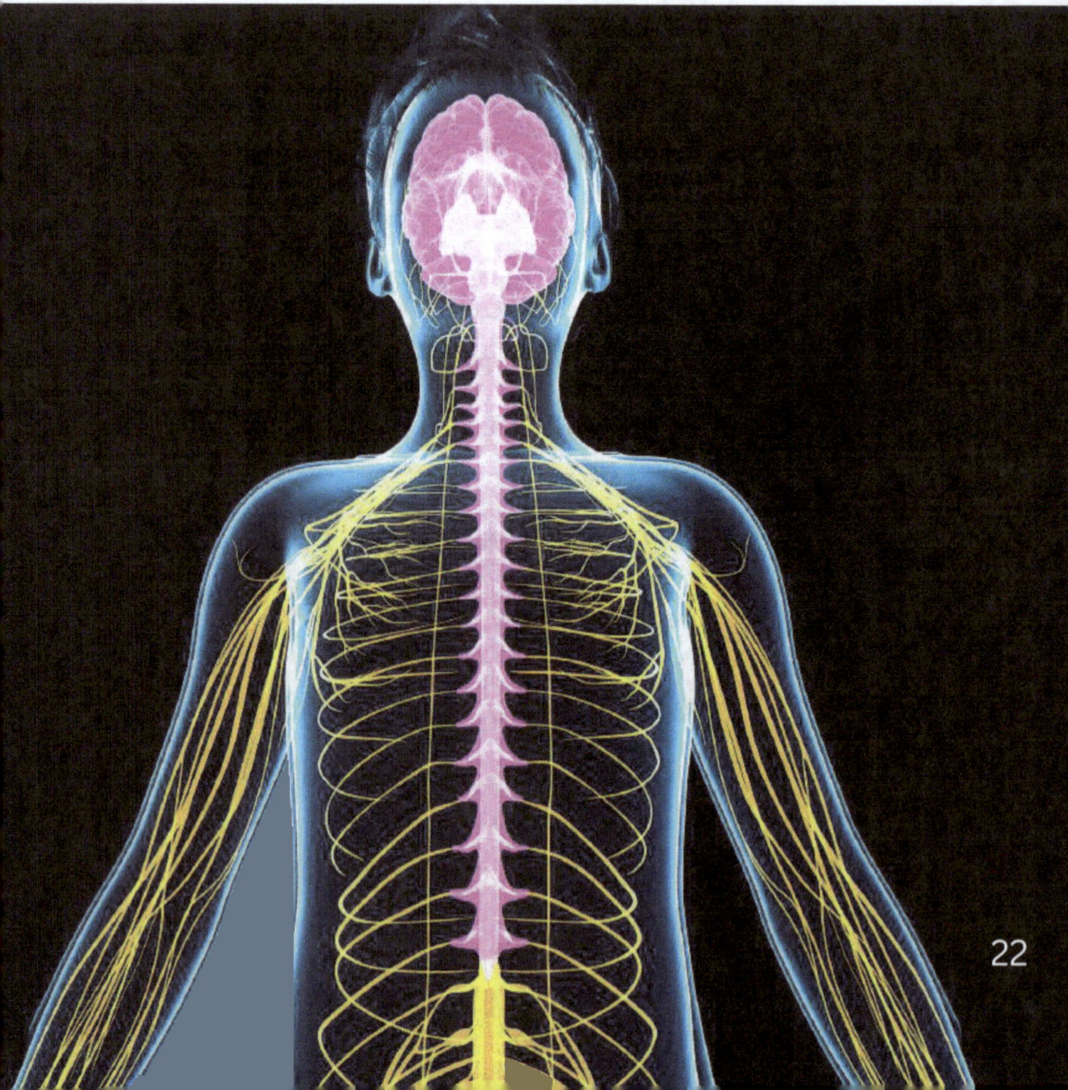

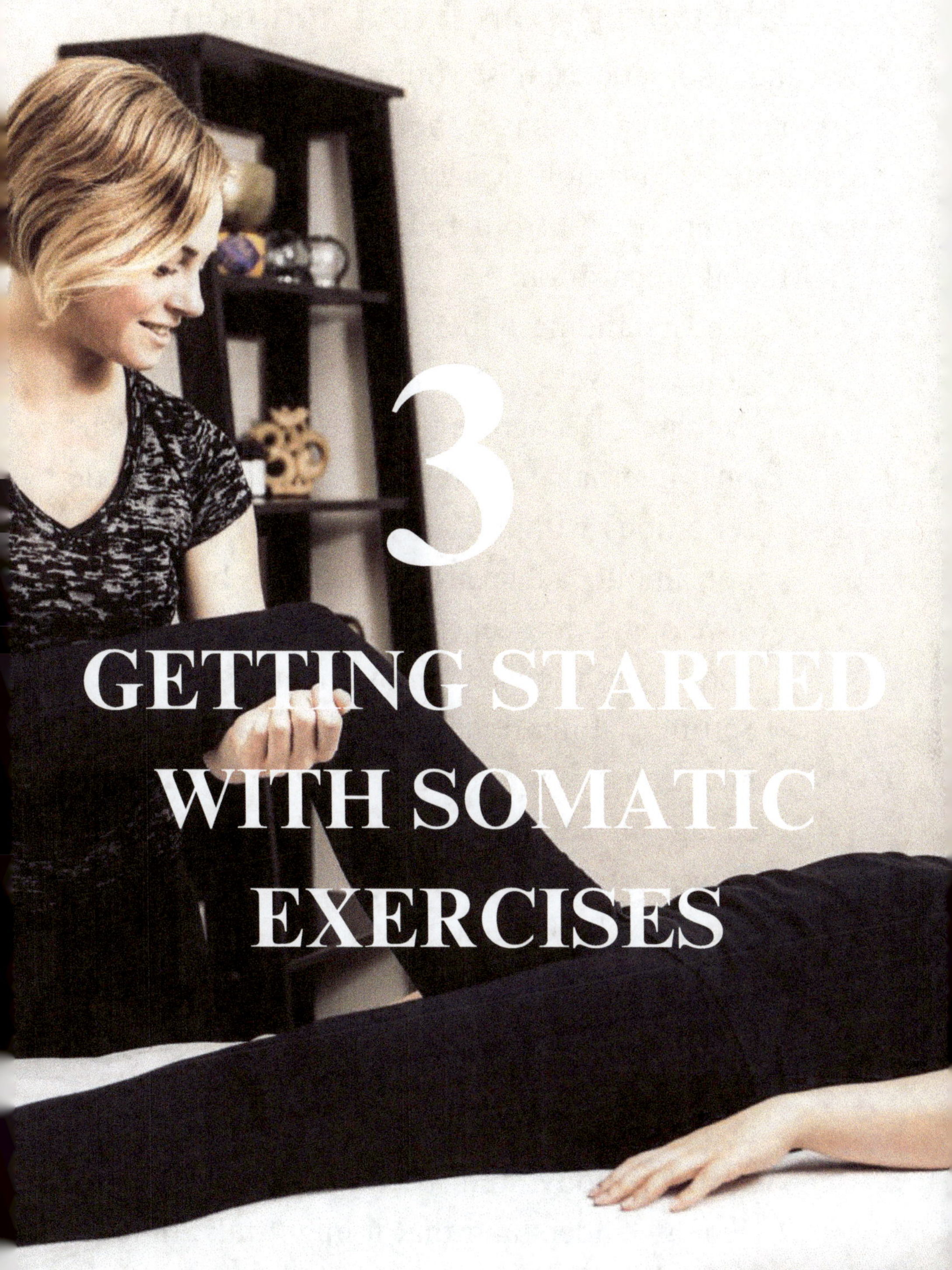

3

GETTING STARTED WITH SOMATIC EXERCISES

Preparing Your Mind and Body

Starting a somatic exercise routine requires a mindful approach that encompasses both mental and physical preparation. This holistic method ensures you derive the maximum benefit from your practice.

1. Mental Preparation:

   - Understanding the Concept: Familiarize yourself with the principles of somatic exercises. Recognize that these exercises focus on internal awareness and the subtle sensations within your body. This practice is not about achieving perfection but about developing a deeper connection with your bodily sensations and movements.

   - Setting Intentions: Begin with clear intentions. Ask yourself why you want to engage in somatic exercises. Whether it's to reduce stress, alleviate pain, or enhance overall well-being, having a clear purpose will guide your practice and keep you motivated.

   - Cultivating Patience: Somatic exercises are about gradual progress and subtle changes. Be patient with yourself as you learn to listen to your body and become attuned to its signals. Understand that it might take time to notice significant changes.

- Mindfulness Practice: Incorporate mindfulness techniques such as deep breathing or meditation to center your mind before beginning your exercises. This helps create a state of calm and focus, allowing you to fully immerse yourself in the practice.

1. Physical Preparation:

   - Body Awareness: Spend a few minutes each day tuning into your body. Notice areas of tension, discomfort, or ease. This practice of body scanning helps you become more aware of your physical state and prepares you for somatic exercises.

   - Hydration and Nutrition: Ensure you are well-hydrated and have eaten adequately. Dehydration and hunger can distract you and affect your concentration during the exercises.

   - Gentle Warm-Up: Engage in a gentle warm-up routine to prepare your muscles and joints. Simple stretches or light movements can help increase blood flow and reduce the risk of injury.

Essential Tools and Equipment

While somatic exercises primarily rely on body awareness and mindful movements, certain tools and equipment can enhance your practice and provide additional support.

1. Comfortable Clothing:
   - Wear loose, comfortable clothing that allows for a full range of motion. Avoid restrictive or tight-fitting garments that might hinder your movements or cause discomfort.

2. Exercise Mat:
   - An exercise mat provides a cushioned surface for floor-based movements, protecting your joints and offering comfort during exercises. Choose a mat with adequate thickness and grip to prevent slipping.

3. Props and Supports:
   - Pillows and Bolsters: These can be used to support various parts of your body, providing comfort and stability during exercises.
   - Yoga Blocks: Useful for maintaining proper alignment and modifying poses to suit your flexibility level.
   - Straps: Assist in stretching and maintaining poses without straining.

4. Calming Aids:
   - Essential Oils: Scents like lavender or chamomile can create a relaxing environment.

Soft Lighting: Dim lighting can enhance relaxation and help you focus on your internal sensations.

- Soothing Music: Gentle, instrumental music or nature sounds can provide a calming backdrop for your practice.

5. Journaling Materials:

- Keeping a journal to record your experiences, sensations, and progress can be an invaluable tool. Reflecting on your practice helps you track your development and identify areas that need attention.

Creating a Calm and Safe Environment

The environment in which you practice somatic exercises significantly impacts your experience. Creating a calm, safe, and welcoming space allows you to fully engage with your practice and derive maximum benefits.

1. Choose the Right Space:

- Select a quiet, clutter-free area where you won't be disturbed. This could be a dedicated room, a corner of your living room, or even an outdoor space where you feel comfortable and relaxed.

2. Set the Atmosphere:

- Lighting: Soft, natural lighting is ideal. If practicing in the evening, use dim lights or candles to create a soothing ambiance.

- Temperature: Ensure the room temperature is comfortable. Too hot or too cold can distract you from focusing on your movements and sensations.
  - Sound: Minimize external noises. You might want to use noise-canceling headphones or play calming background music to help you concentrate.

3. Personalize Your Space:
  - Decorate with items that promote a sense of peace and relaxation. This could include plants, artwork, or personal mementos that make you feel grounded and at ease.

4. Safety Considerations:
  - Ensure that the floor is free from obstacles or hazards that could cause injury. If you're practicing on a hard surface, use a mat to cushion your movements.

5. Detox:
  - Turn off or silence electronic devices to avoid interruptions. Consider using a dedicated device for any guided sessions to prevent distractions from notifications or calls.

Setting Realistic Goals

Setting realistic and achievable goals is crucial for maintaining motivation and ensuring long-term success in your somatic exercise practice. These goals will guide your journey and provide a sense of direction and accomplishment.

1. Define Your Objectives:
   - Clearly outline what you hope to achieve through somatic exercises. Your goals might include reducing stress, managing chronic pain, improving body awareness, or enhancing overall well-being.

2. Break Down Your Goals:
   - Divide your main objectives into smaller, manageable steps. For example, if your goal is to reduce stress, you might start with a daily five-minute breathing exercise, gradually increasing the duration and complexity of your practice.

3. Set SMART Goals:
   - Ensure your goals are Specific, Measurable, Achievable, Relevant, and Time-bound (SMART). This approach provides clarity and structure, making it easier to track your progress and stay motivated.

4. Create a Routine:
   - Establish a regular practice schedule that fits into your daily life. Consistency is key to experiencing the benefits of somatic exercises. Start with shorter sessions and gradually increase the duration as you become more comfortable.
5. Be Flexible:
   - While having a routine is important, it's equally crucial to remain flexible and adaptable. Life can be unpredictable, and there may be days when sticking to your schedule is challenging. Allow yourself the grace to modify your routine as needed without feeling guilty.
6. Track Your Progress:
   - Keep a journal or use a digital app to record your experiences, sensations, and achievements. Reflecting on your journey helps you stay motivated and recognize the progress you've made, no matter how small.
7. Celebrate Milestones:
   - Acknowledge and celebrate your achievements along the way. This could be as simple as taking a moment to appreciate your dedication or treating yourself to a relaxing activity you enjoy.

8. Seek Support:

- Consider joining a class or finding a practice partner to stay motivated. Sharing your journey with others can provide encouragement, accountability, and a sense of community.

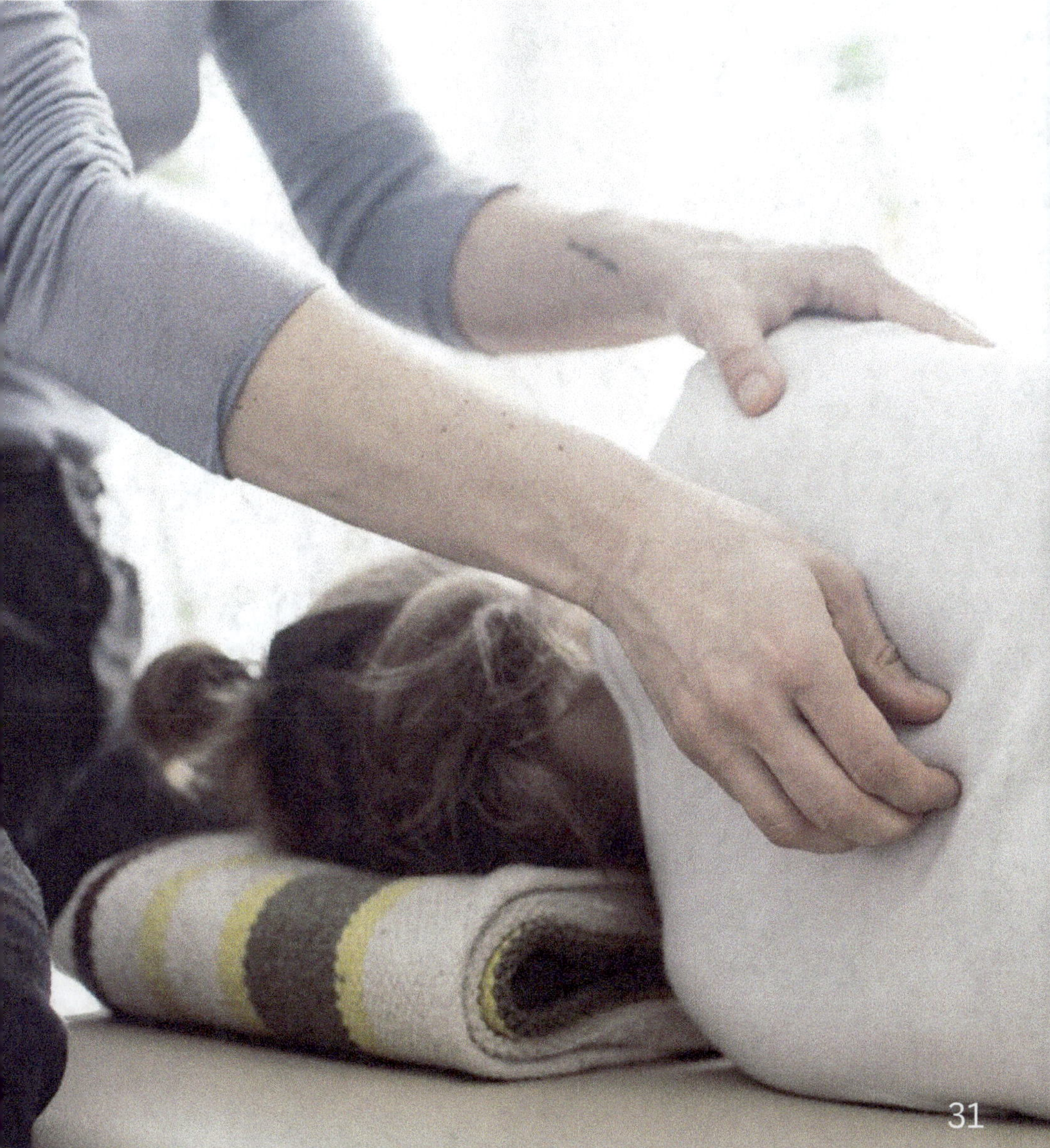

4

DAILY SOMATIC PRACTICES FOR STRESS RELIEF

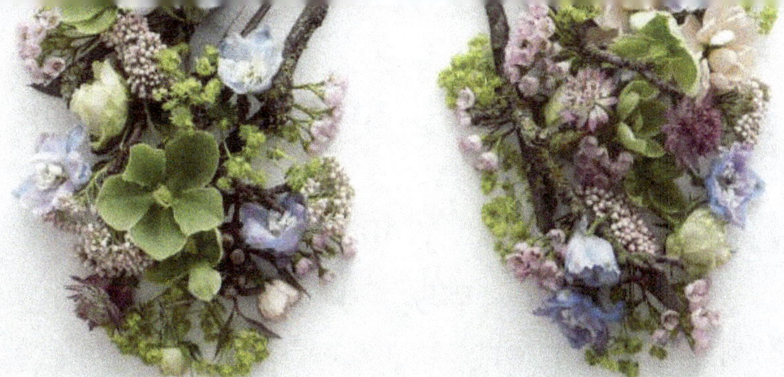

Daily somatic practices can be a powerful tool for managing stress and promoting overall well-being. By incorporating simple exercises into your routine, you can maintain a balanced nervous system, reduce tension, and achieve a sense of relaxation throughout your day. This chapter provides practical guidance on integrating somatic practices into your morning, midday, and evening routines, along with guided techniques for daily stress relief.

Simple Exercises to Start Your Day

Starting your day with somatic exercises can set a positive tone, preparing your mind and body for the challenges ahead. Here are some simple exercises to help you begin your day with calm and focus:

1. Morning Body Scan:
    - Purpose: Increase body awareness and identify areas of tension.
    - How to Perform:
        - Lie on your back or sit comfortably with your eyes closed.

- Take a few deep breaths, allowing your body to relax.
        - Slowly scan your body from head to toe, noticing any areas of tension or discomfort.
        - Acknowledge these areas without judgment and breathe into them, imagining the tension melting away.
    - Duration: 5-10 minutes.

2. Cat-Cow Stretch:
    - Purpose: Mobilize the spine and release tension in the back.
    - How to Perform:
        - Start on your hands and knees in a tabletop position.
        - Inhale as you arch your back, lifting your head and tailbone towards the ceiling (Cow Pose).
        - Exhale as you round your spine, tucking your chin and tailbone (Cat Pose).
        - Repeat the movements, synchronizing with your breath.
    - Duration: 5 minutes.

3. Seated Forward Bend:
    - Purpose: Stretch the hamstrings and lower back, promoting relaxation.
    - How to Perform:

- Sit on the floor with your legs extended in front of you.
- Inhale and lengthen your spine.
- Exhale and hinge at your hips, reaching for your feet or shins.
- Hold the position, breathing deeply and relaxing into the stretch.
  - Duration: 3-5 minutes.

4. Breath Awareness:
  - Purpose: Center your mind and prepare for the day.
  - How to Perform:
    - Sit or lie down comfortably with your eyes closed.
    - Place one hand on your chest and the other on your abdomen.
    - Take slow, deep breaths, feeling your abdomen rise and fall.
    - Focus on the rhythm of your breath, letting go of any distractions.

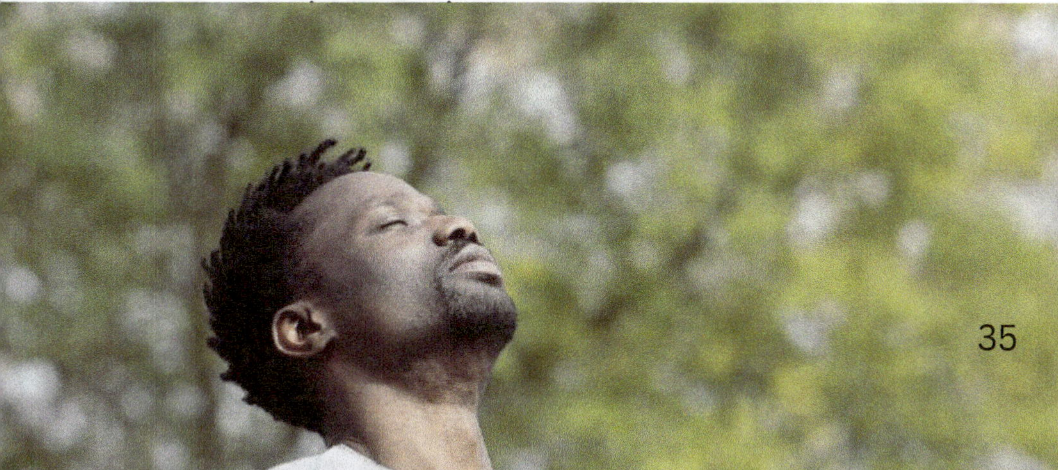

Evening Routines for Relaxation

Ending your day with somatic practices can help you unwind, release accumulated stress, and prepare for restful sleep. Incorporate these evening routines to enhance relaxation and promote a sense of calm:

1. Legs-Up-the-Wall Pose:
   - Purpose: Relax the lower body and promote circulation.
   - How to Perform:
     - Sit with one hip against a wall and swing your legs up, lying down with your back on the floor.
     - Adjust your distance from the wall so that your legs are comfortably resting against it.
     - Close your eyes and take slow, deep breaths, allowing your body to relax.
   - Duration: 5-10 minutes.
2. Child's Pose:
   - Purpose: Stretch the back and relax the mind.
   - How to Perform:
     - Start on your hands and knees, then sit back on your heels and stretch your arms forward, resting your forehead on the floor.

  - Breathe deeply, allowing your body to relax into the pose.
- Duration: 5 minutes.

3. Gentle Neck Stretches:
- Purpose: Release tension in the neck and shoulders.
- How to Perform:
  - Sit or stand with your back straight.
  - Gently tilt your head to one side, bringing your ear towards your shoulder.
  - Hold the stretch, breathing deeply, then switch sides.
  - You can also gently roll your head in a circular motion to release tension.
- Duration: 2-3 minutes each side.

4. Progressive Muscle Relaxation:
- Purpose: Reduce muscle tension and promote overall relaxation.
- How to Perform:
  - Lie down in a comfortable position.
  - Starting with your feet, tense the muscles for a few seconds, then release and relax.
  - Gradually move up through your body, tensing and relaxing each muscle group.
  - Focus on the sensations of tension and relaxation, breathing deeply throughout the process.

Guided Techniques for Daily Relief

Guided techniques can provide structured support for your somatic practice, helping you achieve deeper relaxation and stress relief. Here are some guided practices you can incorporate into your daily routine:

1. Guided Body Scan Meditation:
   - Purpose: Increase body awareness and promote relaxation.
   - How to Perform:
     - Find a comfortable position, either lying down or seated.
     - Close your eyes and take a few deep breaths.
     - Starting at your toes, slowly guide your attention through each part of your body, noticing any sensations or areas of tension.
     - Breathe into these areas, allowing them to relax and release.
     - Continue moving through your body, up to the top of your head.
   - Duration: 15-20 minutes.

2. Breathing Visualization:
- Purpose: Enhance relaxation and reduce stress.
- How to Perform:
    - Sit or lie down comfortably and close your eyes.
    - Take a few deep breaths to center yourself.
    - Visualize a calming scene, such as a beach or a forest.
    - As you breathe in, imagine drawing in the calm and serenity of this scene.
    - As you breathe out, visualize releasing any tension or stress.
    - Continue this visualization, allowing yourself to fully immerse in the peaceful imagery.
- Duration: 10-15 minutes.

3. Mindful Movement Sequence:
- Purpose: Connect with your body and release tension through gentle movement.
- How to Perform:
    - Find a quiet space where you can move freely.
    - Close your eyes and take a few deep breaths.
    - Begin to move your body slowly and mindfully, following your intuition.
    - Focus on the sensations of each movement, staying present and aware.
    - Incorporate stretches, gentle twists, and fluid

- motions that feel good for your body.
    - Allow yourself to move freely and expressively, without judgment or expectation.
  - Duration: 15-20 minutes.

4. Loving-Kindness Meditation:
    - Purpose: Cultivate compassion and reduce emotional stress.
    - How to Perform:
    - Sit comfortably with your eyes closed.
    - Take a few deep breaths to center yourself.
    - Begin by focusing on yourself, silently repeating phrases of loving-kindness, such as "May I be happy, may I be healthy, may I be at peace."
    - Gradually expand your focus to include others, starting with loved ones and eventually extending to all beings.
    - Repeat the phrases, visualizing each person or group and sending them feelings of love and compassion.
    - Duration: 10-15 minutes.

Conclusion

Incorporating daily somatic practices for stress relief into your routine can transform your overall well-being. By starting your day with mindful exercises, incorporating midday practices to reduce tension, and ending with evening routines for relaxation, you create a comprehensive approach to managing stress.

Guided techniques provide additional support, helping you deepen your practice and achieve greater levels of calm and balance. Remember, consistency is key, and each small step you take contributes to a healthier, more relaxed you.

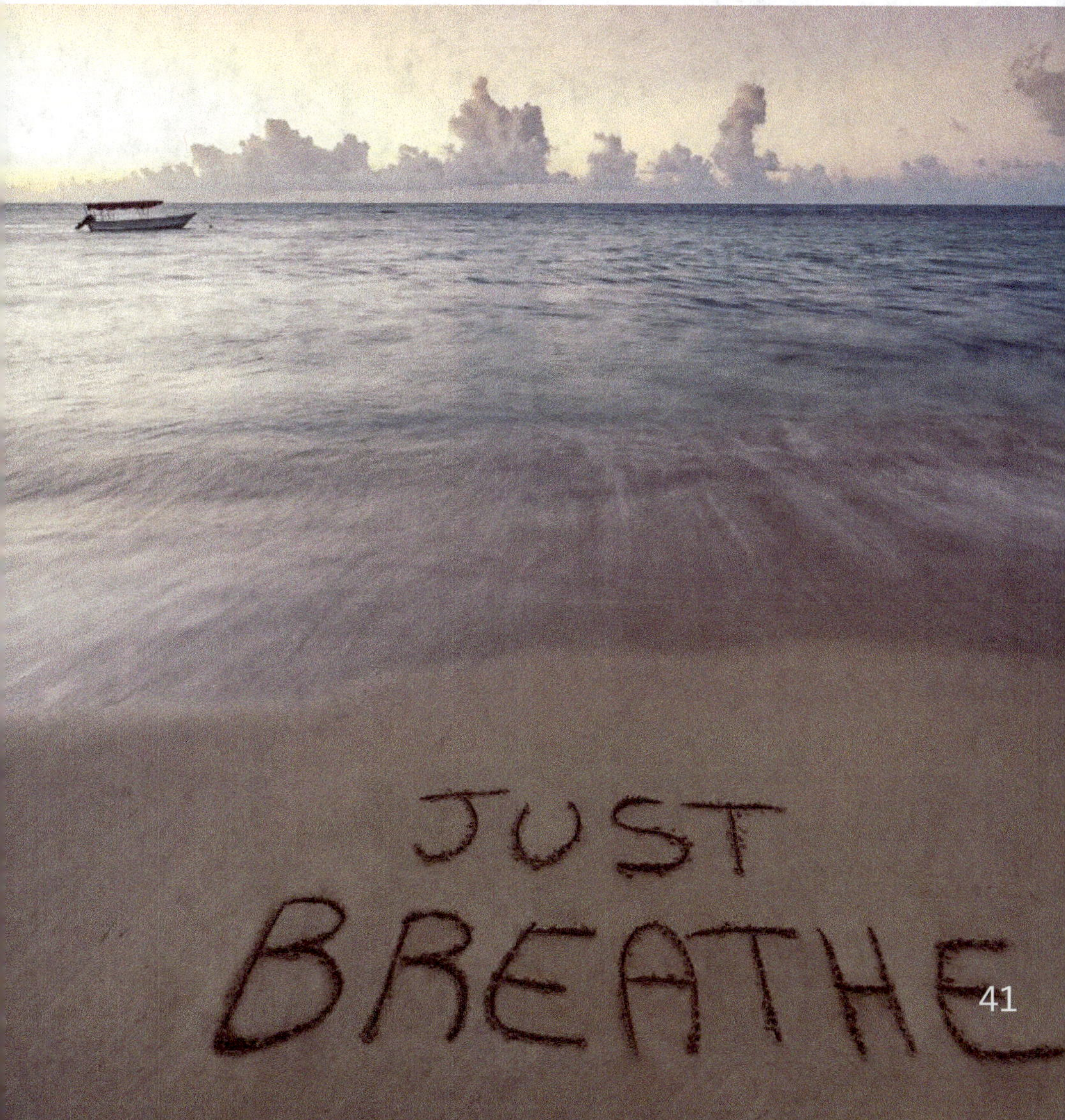

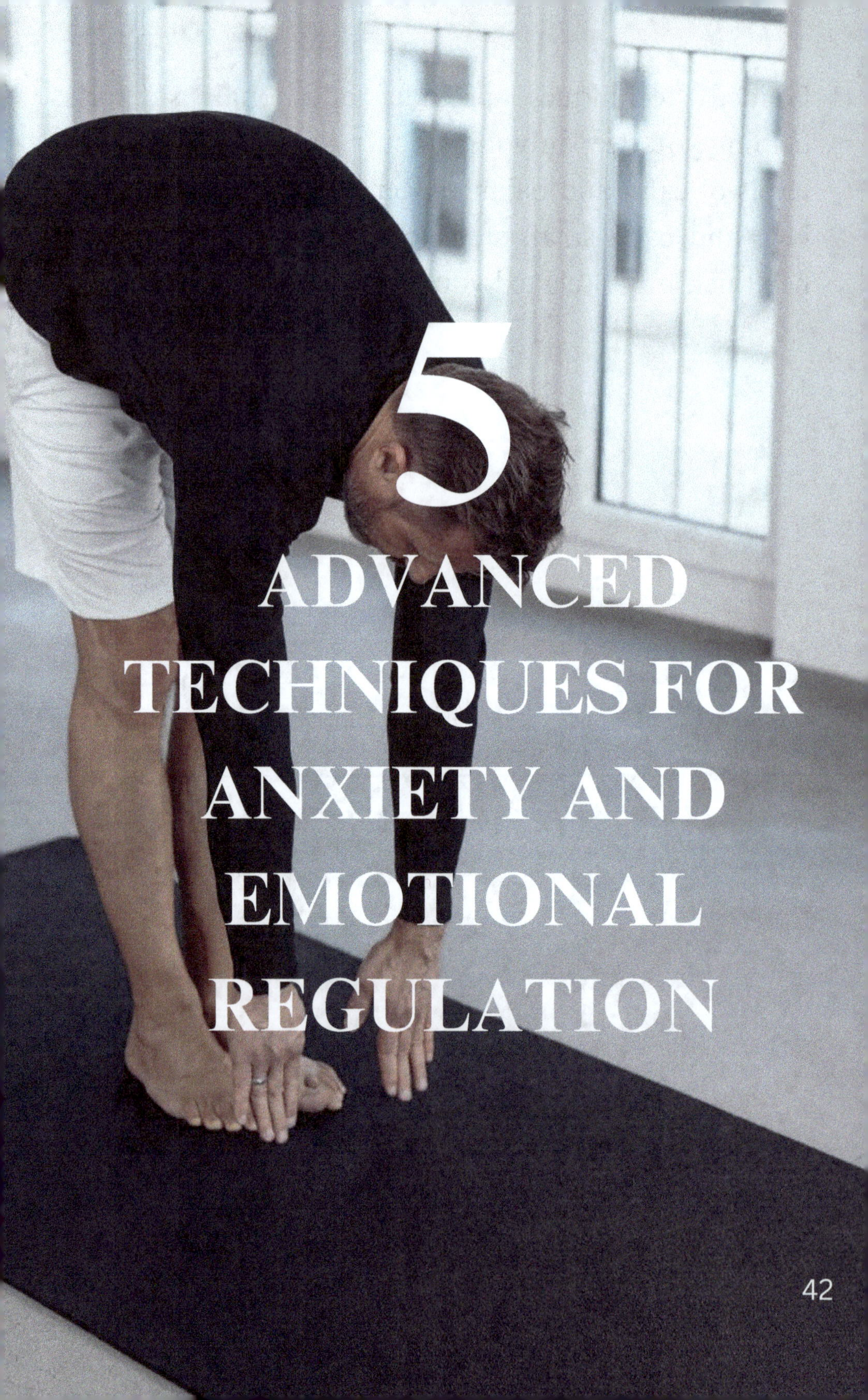

5

ADVANCED TECHNIQUES FOR ANXIETY AND EMOTIONAL REGULATION

As you progress in your somatic practice, incorporating advanced techniques can further enhance your ability to manage anxiety and regulate your emotions. This chapter will delve into specialized breathing exercises, movement practices, mindfulness and meditation techniques, and strategies for integrating these advanced methods into your daily routine for optimal emotional balance and well-being.

Breathing Exercises for Anxiety Reduction

Breathing exercises are powerful tools for reducing anxiety and promoting a sense of calm. These advanced techniques focus on deep, controlled breathing to regulate the nervous system and alleviate stress.

1. 4-7-8 Breathing Technique:
   - Purpose: Promote relaxation and reduce anxiety.
   - How to Perform:
     - Sit or lie down comfortably with your back straight.
     - Close your eyes and take a deep breath in through your nose for a count of 4.
     - Hold your breath for a count of 7.
     - Exhale slowly through your mouth for a count of 8.

- Repeat the cycle 4-8 times, focusing on the rhythm of your breath.
  - Duration: 5-10 minutes.

2. Diaphragmatic Breathing:
- Purpose: Activate the diaphragm for deeper, more efficient breathing and anxiety reduction.
- How to Perform:
  - Lie on your back with one hand on your chest and the other on your abdomen.
  - Take a deep breath in through your nose, allowing your abdomen to rise while keeping your chest still.
  - Exhale slowly through your mouth, feeling your abdomen fall.
  - Focus on breathing deeply into your diaphragm, rather than shallow chest breathing.
- Duration: 10-15 minutes.

3. Alternate Nostril Breathing (Nadi Shodhana):
- Purpose: Balance the nervous system and reduce anxiety.
- How to Perform:
  - Sit comfortably with your spine straight and shoulders relaxed.
  - Use your right thumb to close your right nostril.

- Inhale deeply through your left nostril.
    - Close your left nostril with your right ring finger and release your right nostril.
    - Exhale slowly through your right nostril.
    - Inhale deeply through your right nostril, then close it with your right thumb.
    - Release your left nostril and exhale slowly through your left nostril.
    - Continue alternating for several breaths.
    - Duration: 5-10 minutes

4. Box Breathing (Square Breathing):
  - Purpose: Calm the mind and body by focusing on breath control.
  - How to Perform:
    - Sit comfortably with your back straight and hands resting on your lap.
    - Inhale deeply through your nose for a count of 4.
    - Hold your breath for a count of 4.
    - Exhale slowly through your mouth for a count of 4.
    - Hold your breath for a count of 4.
    - Repeat the cycle for several minutes, maintaining a steady rhythm.
  - Duration: 5-10 minutes.

Movement Practices to Release Emotional Trauma

Movement practices can help release stored emotional trauma and facilitate emotional regulation. These advanced techniques combine mindful movement with somatic awareness to promote healing and balance.

1. Somatic Shaking:
    - Purpose: Release physical and emotional tension stored in the body.
    - How to Perform:
        - Stand with your feet shoulder-width apart and knees slightly bent.
        - Close your eyes and take a few deep breaths.
        - Begin to shake your body gently, starting from your feet and gradually moving up to your head.
        - Allow your body to shake naturally, without forcing or controlling the movement.
        - Continue shaking for several minutes, then gradually slow down and come to stillness.
        - Take a few deep breaths and notice how your body feels.

2. **Mindful Dance:**
    - Purpose: Express and release emotions through free-form movement.
    - How to Perform:
        - Find a space where you can move freely and comfortably.
        - Put on music that resonates with you emotionally.
        - Close your eyes and allow your body to move to the rhythm of the music.
        - Focus on the sensations in your body and let your movements be guided by your emotions.
        - Dance for as long as you feel comfortable, then take a moment to reflect on your experience.
    - Duration: 10-20 minutes.
3. **Yoga for Emotional Release:**
    - Purpose: Use yoga postures to release emotional tension and promote relaxation.
    - How to Perform:
        - Begin with a gentle warm-up to prepare your body.
        - Practice a series of yoga postures that focus on opening the hips, chest, and shoulders, such as Pigeon Pose, Camel Pose, and Child's Pose.

- Hold each posture for several breaths, allowing your body to relax and release tension.
  - Finish with a restorative posture, such as Savasana (Corpse Pose), and take a few minutes to breathe deeply and relax.
- Duration: 20-30 minutes.

Mindfulness and Meditation for Emotional Balance

Mindfulness and meditation practices can help you achieve emotional balance by fostering awareness, acceptance, and compassion. These techniques are essential for managing anxiety and regulating emotions.

1. Loving-Kindness Meditation:
   - Purpose: Cultivate compassion and reduce emotional stress.
   - How to Perform:
     - Sit comfortably with your eyes closed.
     - Take a few deep breaths to center yourself.
     - Begin by focusing on yourself, silently repeating phrases of loving-kindness, such as "May I be happy, may I be healthy, may I be at peace.

- Gradually expand your focus to include others, starting with loved ones and eventually extending to all beings.
- Repeat the phrases, visualizing each person or group and sending them feelings of love and compassion.
- Duration: 10-15 minutes.

2. Mindful Breathing:
- Purpose: Anchor yourself in the present moment and reduce anxiety.
- How to Perform:
  - Sit or lie down comfortably and close your eyes.
  - Focus on your breath, noticing the sensation of air entering and leaving your nostrils.
  - If your mind wanders, gently bring your focus back to your breath.
  - Continue observing your breath, staying present and aware.
  - Duration: 10-15 minutes.

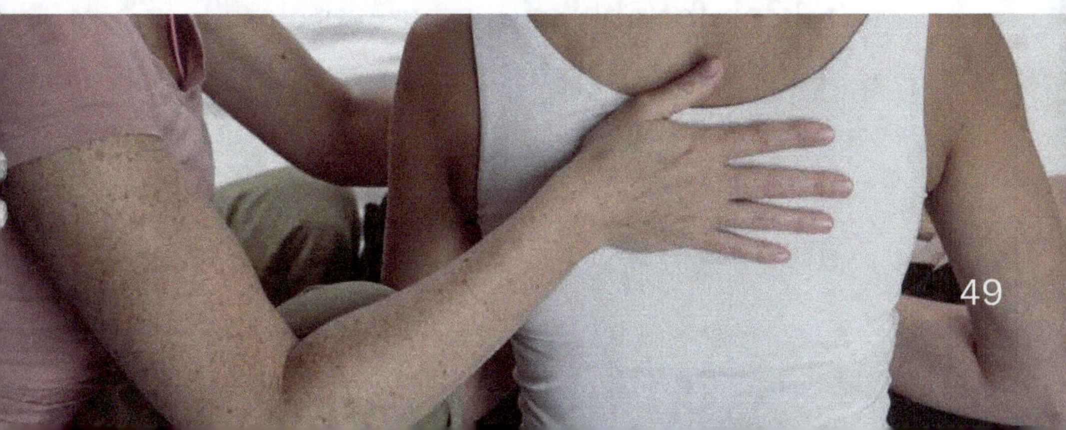

3. Body Scan Meditation:
   - Purpose: Increase body awareness and promote relaxation.
   - How to Perform:
     - Find a comfortable position, either lying down or seated.
     - Close your eyes and take a few deep breaths.
     - Starting at your toes, slowly guide your attention through each part of your body, noticing any sensations or areas of tension.
     - Breathe into these areas, allowing them to relax and release.
     - Continue moving through your body, up to the top of your head.
     - Duration: 15-20 minutes.

4. Mindfulness of Emotions:
   - Purpose: Develop awareness and acceptance of your emotional states.
   - How to Perform:
     - Sit comfortably with your eyes closed.
     - Take a few deep breaths to center yourself.
     - Bring your attention to your current emotional state, noticing any feelings that arise.

- Observe your emotions without judgment, simply acknowledging their presence.
- Use phrases such as "I notice that I am feeling…" to describe your emotions.
- Breathe deeply, allowing yourself to experience and accept each emotion.
- Duration: 10-15 minutes.

Integrating Advanced Techniques into Your Routine

Integrating these advanced somatic techniques into your daily routine can be transformative for your emotional well-being. Here are some strategies to help you incorporate these practices seamlessly:

1. Create a Schedule:
   - Designate specific times each day for your somatic practices.
   - Consistency is key, so try to practice at the same times each day.
2. Mix and Match:
   - Combine different techniques to suit your needs and preferences.
   - For example, you might start your day with diaphragmatic breathing, take a mindful walking break at midday, and end with a body scan meditation in the evening.

- Hold each posture for several breaths, allowing your body to relax and release tension.
    - Finish with a restorative posture, such as Savasana (Corpse Pose), and take a few minutes to breathe deeply and relax.
  - Duration: 20-30 minutes.

3. Listen to Your Body:
  - Pay attention to how your body and emotions respond to different practices.
  - Adjust your routine as needed, focusing on techniques that provide the most benefit.

4. Use Technology:
    - Utilize apps, online videos, and guided meditations to support your practice.
    - These resources can provide structure and guidance, making it easier to stay consistent.

5. Join a Community:
    - Consider joining a somatic practice group or community.
    - Sharing your journey with others can provide motivation, support, and accountability.

6. Set Intentions:
    - Before each practice, set a clear intention for what you hope to achieve.

- This can help you stay focused and motivated, enhancing the effectiveness of your practice.

7. Reflect and Adjust:
    - Regularly reflect on your progress and experiences.
    - Identify what's working well and what could be improved, making adjustments as needed.

Conclusion

Advanced somatic techniques for anxiety and emotional regulation can have a profound impact on your overall well-being. By integrating breathing exercises, movement practices, mindfulness, and meditation into your routine, you can achieve greater emotional balance, reduce anxiety, and heal from past traumas. Remember, the key to success is consistency and a willingness to explore and adapt these practices to your unique needs and experiences.

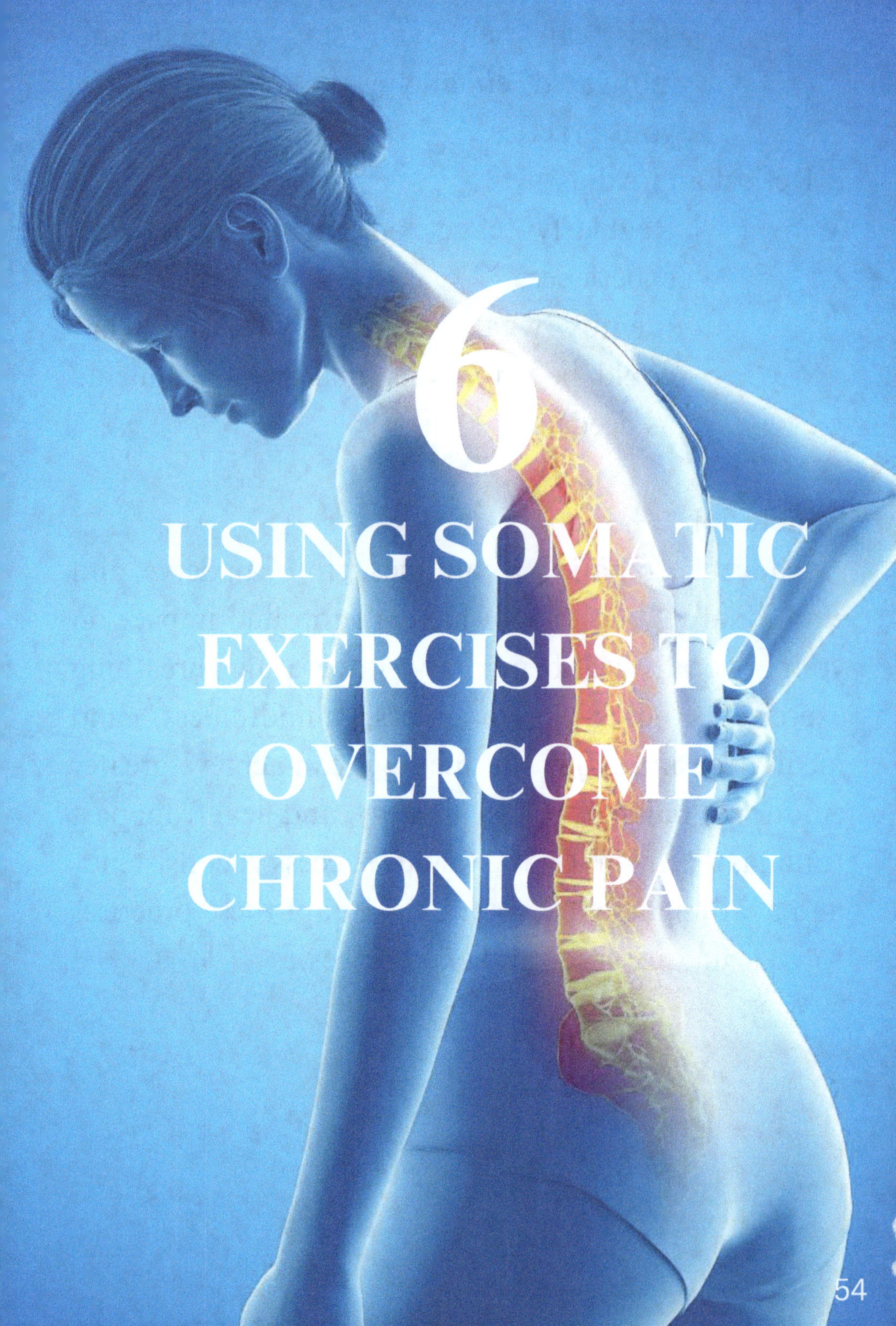

6
USING SOMATIC EXERCISES TO OVERCOME CHRONIC PAIN

Chronic pain is a persistent condition that affects millions of people worldwide. It can significantly impact daily life, causing physical discomfort, emotional distress, and a decrease in quality of life. Somatic exercises offer a holistic approach to managing and alleviating chronic pain by addressing the body-mind connection. In this chapter, we will explore the nature of chronic pain, introduce somatic movements designed for pain relief, discuss techniques for targeting specific pain areas, and provide guidance on developing a comprehensive pain management plan.

Understanding Chronic Pain and Its Triggers

Chronic pain is defined as pain that persists for more than three to six months, beyond the normal healing time. Unlike acute pain, which is a direct response to injury or illness, chronic pain often has complex origins and can be influenced by various physical, emotional, and psychological factors.

1. Physiological Factors:

Nervous System Sensitization: Chronic pain can result from the nervous system becoming overly sensitized to pain signals, a condition known as central sensitization. This can cause even minor stimuli to be perceived as painful..

- Inflammation: Ongoing inflammation in tissues and joints can contribute to persistent pain.
- Muscle Tension and Spasms: Chronic muscle tension and spasms, often resulting from poor posture or repetitive strain, can exacerbate pain

2. Emotional and Psychological Factors:

- Stress and Anxiety: Chronic stress and anxiety can heighten pain perception and contribute to muscle tension.
- Depression: Chronic pain and depression often coexist, with each condition exacerbating the other.
- Trauma: Past physical or emotional trauma can leave lasting imprints on the body, manifesting as chronic pain.

3. Lifestyle Factors:

- Sedentary Lifestyle: Lack of physical activity can weaken muscles and joints, leading to pain.
- Poor Nutrition: Inadequate nutrition can contribute to inflammation and poor tissue health.
- Sleep Deprivation: Poor sleep can reduce the body's ability to heal and increase pain sensitivity.

Somatic Movements for Pain Relief

Somatic movements are gentle, mindful exercises that focus on body awareness and the release of muscle tension. These movements can help reduce chronic pain by retraining the nervous system and improving overall body function.

1. Pandiculation:
   - Purpose: Reset muscle length and tension by mimicking the natural stretching movements of animals.
   - How to Perform:
     - Start by contracting a muscle group slowly and intentionally.
     - Gradually release the contraction while focusing on the sensations in the muscle.
     - Extend the muscle gently, as if stretching after waking up.
     - Repeat for different muscle groups, focusing on areas of tension.
   - Duration: 10-15 minutes daily.
2. Somatic Yoga:
   - Purpose: Combine yoga postures with somatic awareness to relieve tension and improve flexibility.
   - How to Perform:
     - Choose gentle yoga poses that focus on

- stretching and relaxation, such as Child's Pose, Cat-Cow, and Savasana.
    - Perform each pose slowly and mindfully, paying attention to the sensations in your body.
    - Use deep, diaphragmatic breathing to enhance relaxation and release tension.
  - Duration: 20-30 minutes, 3-4 times per week.

3. Body Scanning:
  - Purpose: Increase awareness of areas of tension and pain in the body.
  - How to Perform:
    - Find a comfortable lying or seated position.
    - Close your eyes and take a few deep breaths to center yourself.
    - Starting from your toes, slowly move your attention through each part of your body.
    - Notice any areas of tension, discomfort, or pain without judgment.
    - Breathe into these areas, imagining the tension melting away with each exhale.
  - Duration: 10-15 minutes daily.
4. Gentle Stretching:
  - Purpose: Improve flexibility and reduce

muscle stiffness.

- How to Perform:
    - Identify specific muscle groups that feel tight or sore.
    - Perform gentle stretches for each muscle group, holding each stretch for 20-30 seconds.
    - Avoid bouncing or forcing the stretch; instead, focus on slow, controlled movements.
    - Breathe deeply and evenly throughout the stretches.
- Duration: 10-15 minutes daily.

Techniques to Address Specific Pain Areas

Chronic pain can affect different areas of the body, each requiring tailored techniques for relief. The following somatic exercises target common pain areas, providing specific strategies for alleviating discomfort.

1. Lower Back Pain:
    - Pelvic Tilts:
        - Lie on your back with your knees bent and feet flat on the floor.
        - Gently tilt your pelvis upward, pressing your lower back into the floor.

- - Hold for a few seconds, then release.
    - Repeat 10-15 times, focusing on the movement and sensation in your lower back.
  - Cat-Cow Stretch:
    - Start on your hands and knees in a tabletop position.
    - Inhale as you arch your back (Cow Pose), lifting your head and tailbone.
    - Exhale as you round your back (Cat Pose), tucking your chin and tailbone.
    - Repeat for 1-2 minutes, moving slowly and mindfully.

2. Neck and Shoulder Pain:

- Shoulder Rolls:
  - Sit or stand with your back straight.
  - Roll your shoulders forward in a circular motion, focusing on releasing tension.
  - Repeat 10-15 times, then reverse the direction.
- Neck Stretches:
  - Sit or stand with your back straight.
  - Gently tilt your head to one side, bringing your ear toward your shoulder.
  - Hold for 20-30 seconds, then switch sides.
  - Repeat 2-3 times on each side, breathing deeply.

3. Hip and Knee Pain:
- Hip Circles:
    - Stand with your feet hip-width apart.
    - Place your hands on your hips and gently rotate your hips in a circular motion.
    - Repeat 10-15 times in each direction, focusing on smooth, controlled movements.
- Knee-to-Chest Stretch:
    - Lie on your back with your legs extended.
    - Gently pull one knee toward your chest, holding it with both hands.
    - Hold for 20-30 seconds, then switch legs.
    - Repeat 2-3 times on each side, breathing deeply.

4. Wrist and Hand Pain:
- Wrist Circles:
    - Extend one arm in front of you with your palm facing down.
    - Use your other hand to gently rotate your wrist in a circular motion.
    - Repeat 10-15 times in each direction, then switch hands.
- Finger Stretches:
    - Extend one arm in front of you with your palm facing up.
    - Use your other hand to gently pull back each finger, stretching the muscles and tendons.

Hold for 10-15 seconds per finger, then switch hands.

Developing a Pain Management Plan

Creating a comprehensive pain management plan involves integrating somatic exercises with other strategies to address chronic pain holistically. Here are steps to develop an effective plan:

1. Identify Pain Triggers:
   - Keep a pain diary to track when and where pain occurs, as well as potential triggers such as specific activities, stress, or dietary factors.
2. Set Realistic Goals:
   - Establish short-term and long-term goals for managing pain. Focus on achievable milestones, such as reducing pain intensity or increasing physical activity levels.
3. Incorporate Regular Somatic Practices:
   - Schedule regular somatic exercise sessions, incorporating the movements and techniques discussed earlier. Consistency is key to experiencing long-term benefits.
4. Combine with Other Therapies:
   - Complement somatic exercises with other pain management strategies, such as physical therapy, massage, acupuncture, or counseling. A multidisciplinary approach can enhance results.

5. Monitor Progress:
   - Regularly assess your progress toward your pain management goals. Adjust your plan as needed, based on what is working and what isn't.
6. Prioritize Self-Care:
   - Ensure you are taking care of your overall health and well-being. This includes maintaining a balanced diet, getting enough sleep, managing stress, and staying hydrated.
7. Seek Support:
   - Reach out to healthcare professionals, support groups, or a somatic therapy practitioner for guidance and encouragement. Sharing your journey with others can provide valuable insights and support.

Conclusion

Chronic pain can be a daunting and persistent challenge, but incorporating somatic exercises into your routine offers a powerful and holistic approach to managing and alleviating pain. By understanding the nature of chronic pain, practicing targeted somatic movements, and developing a comprehensive pain management plan, you can regain control over your body and improve your quality of life.

7

SOMATIC EXERCISES FOR OVERALL WELL-BEING

Somatic exercises go beyond mere physical movement —they provide a pathway to enhancing overall well-being by nurturing the mind-body connection, improving emotional resilience, promoting better sleep, and fostering relaxation. This chapter delves into the ways somatic practices contribute to holistic health, offering specific exercises and strategies for integrating these practices into daily life.

Enhancing Your Mind-Body Connection

The mind-body connection is a fundamental aspect of somatic exercises. By cultivating awareness of bodily sensations and integrating this awareness into movement, you can create a harmonious relationship between your mind and body. This connection is vital for overall well-being, as it fosters greater self-awareness, emotional regulation, and physical health.

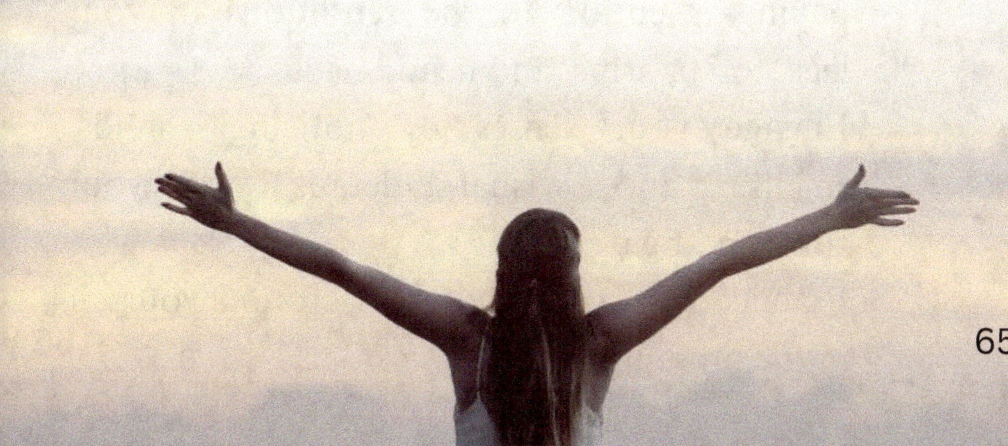

1. Body Awareness Exercises:
- Body Scan Meditation:
    - Find a comfortable position lying down or sitting.
    - Close your eyes and take a few deep breaths.
    - Slowly bring your attention to different parts of your body, starting from your toes and moving upward to your head.
    - Notice any sensations, tension, or discomfort without judgment.
    - Breathe into each area, imagining the tension melting away with each exhale.
    - Practice for 10-15 minutes daily to enhance body awareness.
- Sensory Grounding:
    - Sit or stand comfortably with your feet firmly on the ground.
    - Focus on the sensations in your feet, noticing the connection to the earth.
    - Gradually move your attention upward, paying attention to the sensations in your legs, torso, arms, and head.
    - Engage your senses by noticing sounds, smells, and visual details in your surroundings.
    - Practice for 5-10 minutes to ground yourself in the present moment.

2. Movement with Intention:
- Mindful Walking:
    ◦ Find a quiet space where you can walk without distractions.
    ◦ Walk slowly and deliberately, paying close attention to the sensations in your feet as they touch the ground.
    ◦ Notice the movement of your legs, the rhythm of your breath, and the feeling of your body in motion.
    ◦ Practice for 10-15 minutes, focusing on the present moment and the connection between your mind and body.

Tai Chi or Qigong:
- These ancient practices combine slow, flowing movements with deep breathing and mindfulness.
- Engage in a guided session or follow online tutorials to learn basic movements.
- Practice regularly to enhance the mind-body connection and promote relaxation.

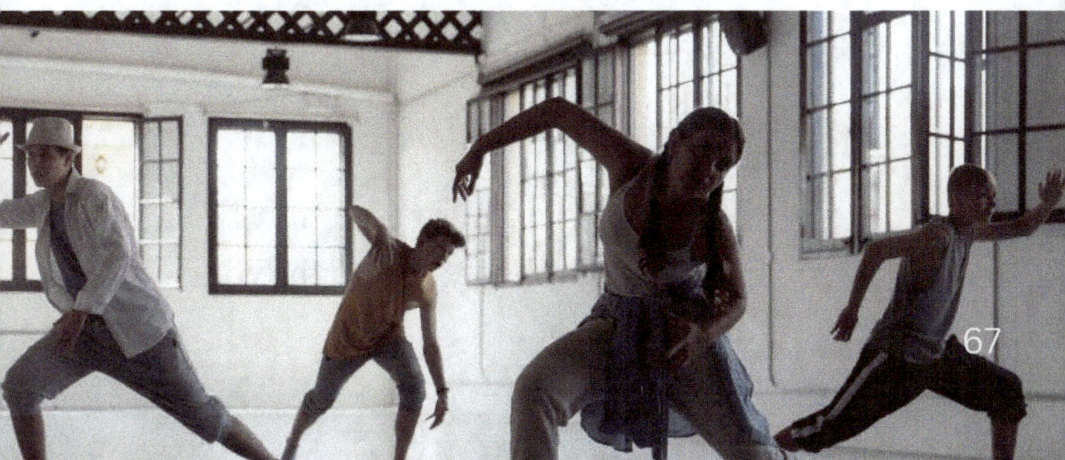

Exercises to Improve Emotional Resilience

Emotional resilience is the ability to adapt to and recover from stress, adversity, and challenging emotions. Somatic exercises can strengthen emotional resilience by promoting self-awareness, regulating the nervous system, and providing tools for emotional expression and release.

1. Breathwork for Emotional Regulation:
   - Diaphragmatic Breathing:
     - Sit or lie down in a comfortable position.
     - Place one hand on your chest and the other on your abdomen.
     - Inhale deeply through your nose, allowing your abdomen to expand while keeping your chest relatively still.
     - Exhale slowly through your mouth, feeling your abdomen contract.
     - Practice for 5-10 minutes to calm the nervous system and regulate emotions.
   - 4-7-8 Breathing:
     - Inhale quietly through your nose for a count of 4.
     - Hold your breath for a count of 7.
     - Exhale completely through your mouth for a count of 8.

Repeat the cycle 4-8 times, focusing on the rhythm of your breath to reduce anxiety and promote emotional balance.

2. Movement for Emotional Expression:
- Shake and Release:
  - Stand with your feet shoulder-width apart and knees slightly bent.
  - Begin to shake your body gently, starting from your feet and moving upward.
  - Gradually increase the intensity of the shaking, allowing your arms, legs, and torso to move freely.
  - Shake for 1-2 minutes, then gradually slow down and come to a still position.
  - Notice any changes in your emotional state and body sensations.
- Dance Therapy:
  - Choose a piece of music that resonates with your current emotional state.
  - Allow your body to move freely and expressively to the rhythm of the music.
  - Focus on the sensations in your body and the emotions that arise.
  - Dance for 5-10 minutes, using movement as a form of emotional release and self-expression.

3. Journaling for Emotional Insight:
- Expressive Writing:

- Set aside 10-15 minutes each day to write about your thoughts and feelings.
  - Write freely without worrying about grammar or structure.
  - Use this time to explore and process your emotions, gaining insight and clarity.
- Gratitude Journaling:
  - Each day, write down three things you are grateful for.
  - Reflect on positive experiences and moments of joy.
  - This practice can shift your focus to positive aspects of your life, enhancing emotional resilience.

Practices for Better Sleep and Relaxation

Quality sleep and relaxation are essential components of overall well-being. Somatic exercises can help regulate the nervous system, reduce stress, and promote restful sleep by creating a state of physical and mental relaxation.

1. Pre-Sleep Relaxation Routine:
   - Progressive Muscle Relaxation:
     - Lie down in a comfortable position.
     - Starting from your toes, tense each muscle group for 5-10 seconds, then release.

Repeat the cycle 4-8 times, focusing on the rhythm of your breath to reduce anxiety and promote emotional balance.

Building a Sustainable Somatic Routine

Creating a sustainable somatic routine involves integrating these practices into your daily life in a way that is manageable and consistent. Here are some strategies to help you build and maintain a routine that supports your overall well-being.

1. Start Small and Gradually Increase:
   - Begin with short, manageable sessions of 5-10 minutes.
   - Gradually increase the duration and complexity of your practices as you become more comfortable and experienced.
2. Create a Schedule:
   - Designate specific times of day for your somatic exercises, such as morning, midday, or evening.
   - Consistency is key—try to practice at the same time each day to establish a routine.
3. Combine with Daily Activities:
   - Integrate somatic exercises into your daily activities, such as mindful walking during your commute or body awareness exercises while sitting at your desk.

o This makes it easier to incorporate somatic practices into your busy schedule.

4. Listen to Your Body:

o Pay attention to how your body feels during and after each practice.

o Adjust your routine based on your body's needs, increasing intensity when you feel capable and reducing it when you need rest.

5. Set Realistic Goals:

o Establish clear, achievable goals for your somatic practice, such as reducing stress, improving sleep, or enhancing emotional resilience.

o Track your progress and celebrate your achievements, no matter how small.

6. Seek Support and Guidance:

o Join a class, workshop, or online community to connect with others who practice somatic exercises.

o Consider working with a somatic therapist or coach to receive personalized guidance and support.

Conclusion

Somatic exercises are powerful tools for enhancing overall well-being by fostering a strong mind-body connection, improving emotional resilience, promoting better sleep, and creating a state of relaxation. By integrating these practices into your daily routine, you can experience profound benefits for your physical, emotional, and mental health. Remember, the key to success is consistency, self-awareness, and a willingness to explore and adapt these practices to your unique needs. Embrace the journey towards holistic well-being, and let somatic exercises guide you towards a balanced, healthy, and fulfilling life.

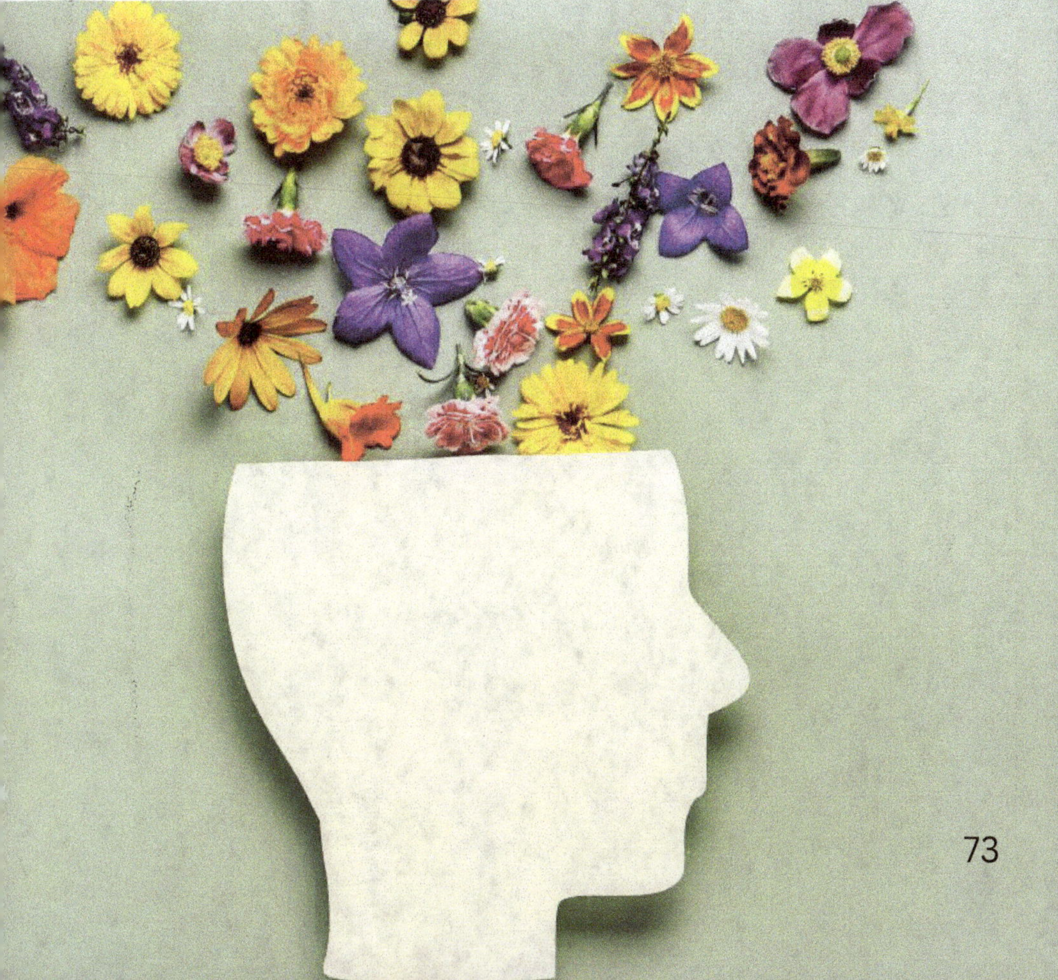

8

PERSONALIZED SOMATIC PLANS AND CASE STUDIES

Creating a personalized somatic exercise plan involves tailoring practices to meet individual needs, goals, and lifestyles. In this chapter, we will explore how to create a personalized plan, share real-life case studies and success stories, discuss strategies for overcoming common challenges, and provide resources for continued learning and support.

Creating a Personalized Somatic Exercise Plan

A personalized somatic exercise plan ensures that the practices align with your specific needs and goals. Here are steps to create an effective plan:

1. Assess Your Needs and Goals:
   - Identify Areas of Focus:
     - Determine the specific areas you want to address, such as stress reduction, anxiety management, pain relief, or emotional regulation.
   - Set Clear Goals:
     - Define what you hope to achieve with your somatic practice. Goals can include improving sleep quality, enhancing emotional resilience, or reducing chronic pain.
2. Choose Appropriate Exercises:

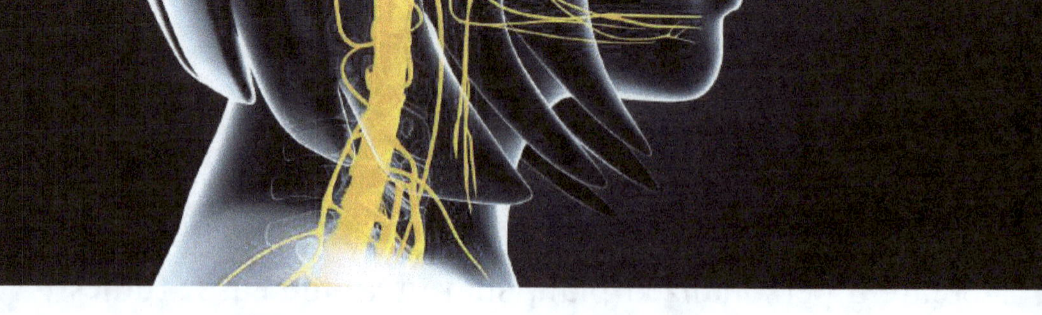

- Select Exercises Based on Goals:
  - Choose somatic exercises that align with your goals. For example, breathing exercises and guided imagery can be effective for stress reduction, while specific movement practices can target chronic pain.
- Balance Variety and Consistency:
  - Incorporate a mix of exercises to keep your routine engaging while maintaining consistency with core practices.

3. Develop a Routine:
  - Schedule Regular Practice:
    - Designate specific times each day for your somatic exercises. Consistency is crucial for long-term benefits.
  - Create a Balanced Routine:
    - Include exercises for different times of the day, such as morning routines to start your day, midday practices for reducing tension, and evening routines for relaxation.

4. Monitor Progress and Adjust:

- Track Your Progress:
  - Keep a journal to record your experiences, noting any changes in your physical, emotional, and mental state.
- Adjust as Needed:
  - Be flexible and adjust your routine based on your progress and any new challenges that arise.

Real-Life Case Studies and Success Stories

Hearing about the experiences of others can be inspiring and provide valuable insights. Here are a few real-life case studies and success stories of individuals who have benefited from somatic exercises:

1. Case Study 1: Sarah's Journey to Overcoming Anxiety
   - Background:
     - Sarah, a 35-year-old marketing professional, struggled with anxiety and panic attacks for years.
   - Somatic Plan:
     - Sarah started with daily breathing exercises and mindfulness meditation. She gradually incorporated gentle

movement practices and body awareness exercises.

- o Results:
    - Within a few months, Sarah noticed a significant reduction in her anxiety levels and fewer panic attacks.
    - She reported improved emotional resilience and a greater sense of calm in her daily life.

2. Case Study 2: John's Path to Managing Chronic Pain

- o Background:
    - John, a 50-year-old construction worker, experienced chronic back pain for over a decade.
- o Somatic Plan:
    - John began with simple stretching exercises and progressive muscle relaxation.
    - He added specific somatic movements targeting his lower back and integrated body awareness practices.
- o Results:
    - John's chronic pain gradually diminished, and he regained mobility and flexibility.
    - He developed a deeper understanding of his body and learned to manage pain effectively through somatic exercises.

3. Case Study 3: Lisa's Transformation Through Emotional Regulation
  - Background:
    - Lisa, a 28-year-old teacher, faced emotional turbulence and difficulty managing stress.
  - Somatic Plan:
    - Lisa engaged in daily journaling, expressive movement, and guided imagery for emotional expression and release.
    - She practiced mindfulness and breathwork to regulate her emotions.
  - Results:
    - Lisa experienced a profound transformation in her emotional resilience and stress management.
    - She reported feeling more balanced, centered, and equipped to handle life's challenges.

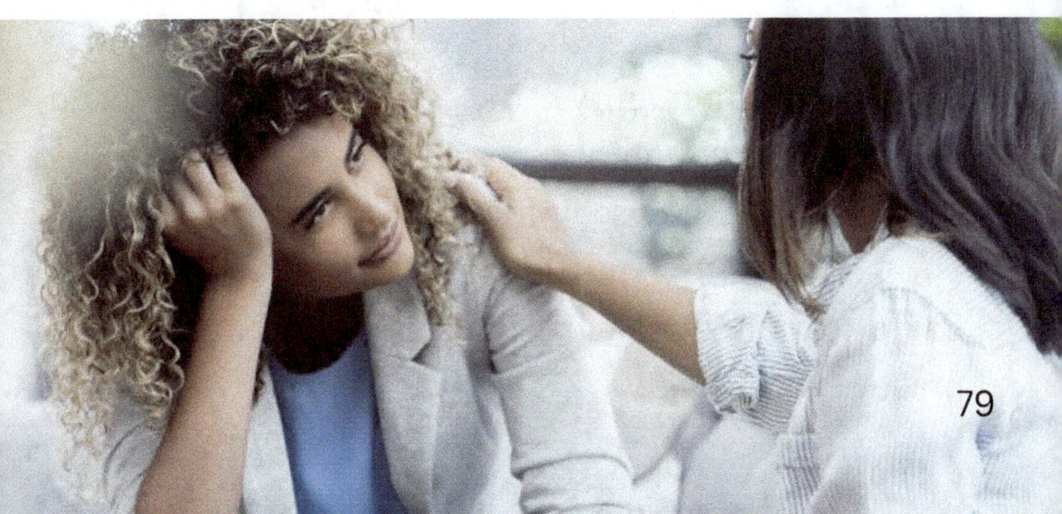

Overcoming Common Challenges

Despite the benefits of somatic exercises, individuals may encounter challenges. Here are strategies to overcome common obstacles:

1. Finding Time for Practice:
   - Integrate into Daily Routine:
     - Combine somatic exercises with daily activities, such as mindful walking during your commute or body awareness exercises while sitting at your desk.
   - Start with Short Sessions:
     - Begin with short, manageable sessions and gradually increase the duration as you become more comfortable.
2. Staying Consistent:
   - Set Reminders:
     - Use alarms or calendar notifications to remind yourself to practice regularly.
   - Accountability:
     - Join a class, workshop, or online community to stay motivated and accountable.
3. Dealing with Discomfort or Resistance:
   - Listen to Your Body:

Pay attention to your body's signals and adjust your practice accordingly.

Avoid pushing through pain or discomfort.

- ○ Seek Support:
    - ▪ Consult with a somatic therapist or coach for guidance and support if you encounter significant challenges.
- Maintaining Motivation:
    - ○ Celebrate Progress:
        - ▪ Acknowledge and celebrate your achievements, no matter how small.
    - ○ Reflect on Benefits:
        - ▪ Regularly reflect on the positive changes and benefits you experience from your somatic practice.

Conclusion

Creating a personalized somatic exercise plan, learning from real-life case studies, overcoming common challenges, and accessing resources for continued learning and support are essential steps toward integrating somatic practices into your life. By doing so, you can experience the profound benefits of somatic exercises for nervous system regulation and overall well-being. Embrace this journey with an open heart and mind, and let the transformative power of somatic practices guide you toward a healthier, more balanced, and fulfilling life.

A Note to My Readers

Thank you for choosing "Somatic Exercises for Nervous System Regulation." Your support means the world to me. If you found this book helpful and enriching, I would be incredibly grateful if you could take a moment to leave a positive review on Amazon. Your feedback not only helps me improve but also assists other readers in discovering the benefits of somatic exercises.

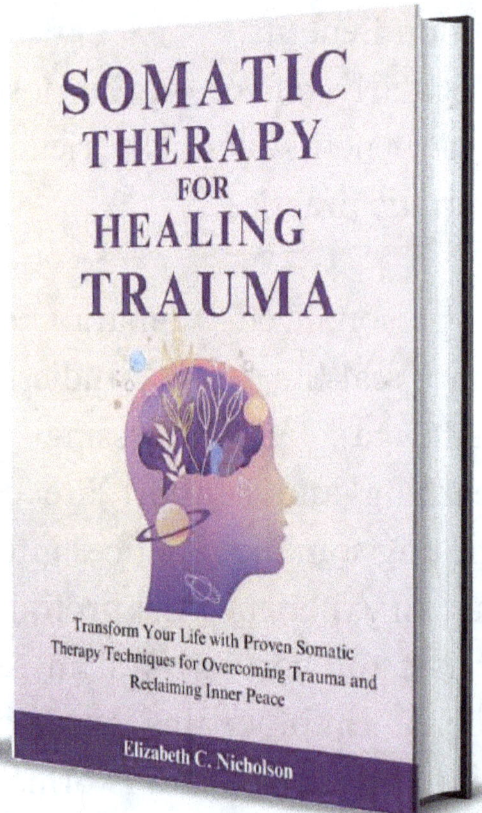

I also invite you to explore another insightful book I've written, "Somatic Therapy for Healing Trauma." This companion book delves deeper into the therapeutic applications of somatic practices specifically designed for trauma recovery. Together, these books provide a comprehensive guide to enhancing your well-being through somatic techniques.

Thank you for being a part of this journey toward better health and well-being.

Warm regards,

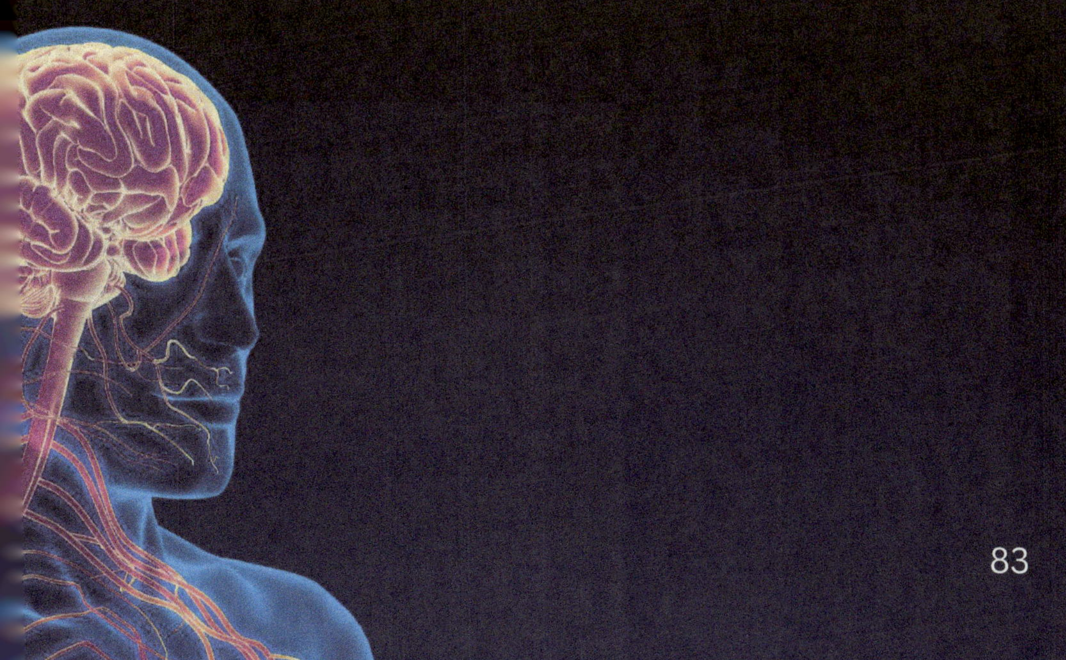

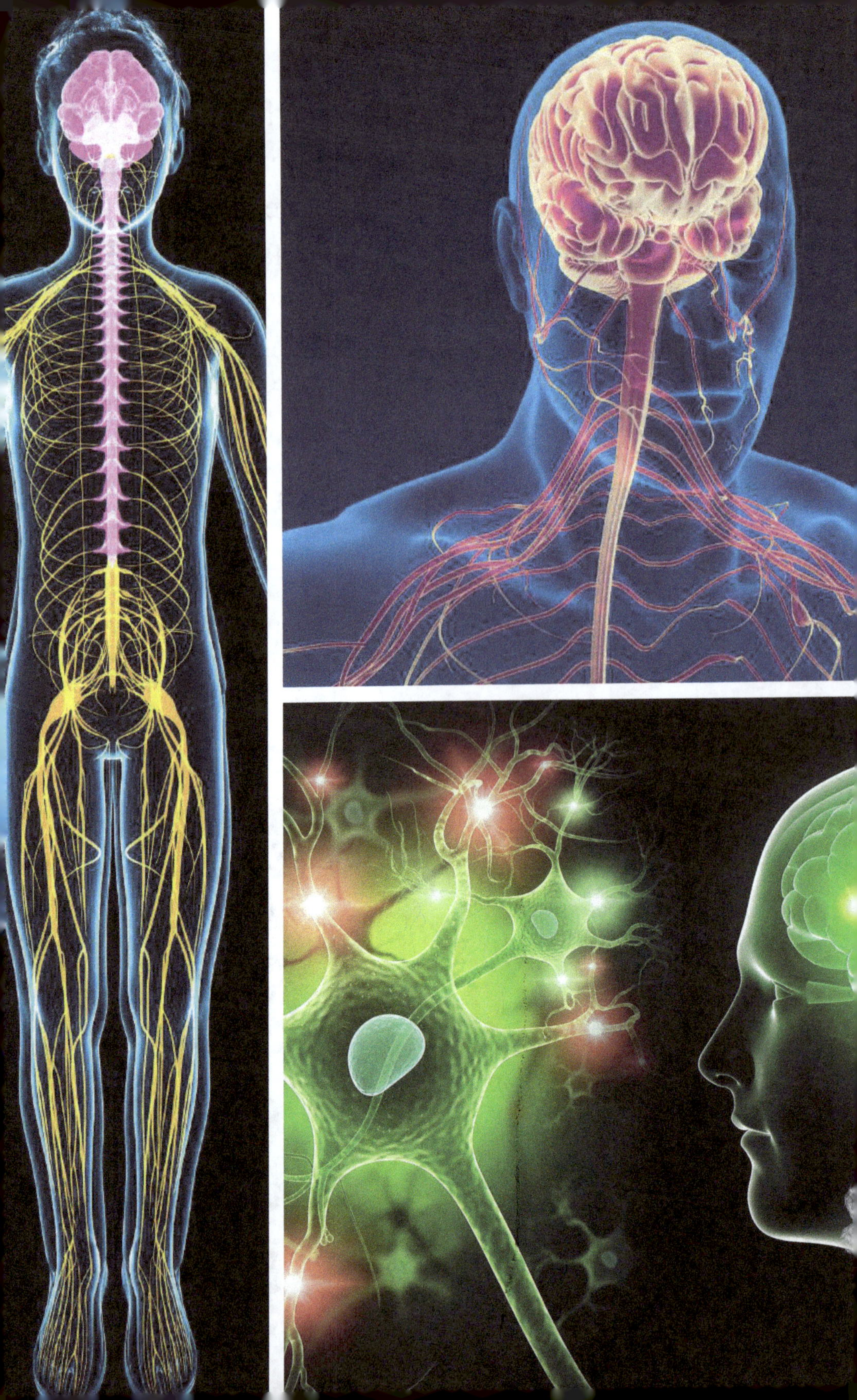